CommunicationLab™

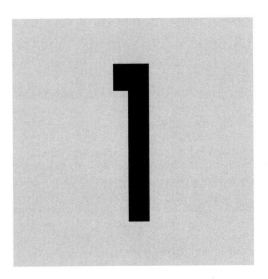

Ellen Pritchard Dodge, M.Ed, CCC-SLP

Skill Area:	Classroom Communication
Ages:	6-14

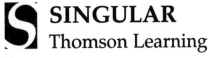
SINGULAR
Thomson Learning

Africa • Australia • Canada • Denmark • Japan • Mexico • New Zealand • Philippines
Puerto Rico • Singapore • Spain • United Kingdom • United States

NOTICE TO THE READER

COPYRIGHT © 1998
Singular Publishing Group is a division of Thomson Learning. The Thomson Learning logo is a registered trademark used herein under license.

Printed in the United States of America
2 3 4 5 6 7 8 9 10 XXX 05 04 03 02 01 00

For more information, contact Singular Publishing Group, 401 West "A" Street, Suite 325 San Diego, CA 92101-7904; or find us on the World Wide Web at http://www.singpub.com

Library of Congress Cataloging-in-Publication Data:
ISBN: 0-769-30006-5

Contents

Preface

In the fields of speech-language pathology and special education, there is a growing recognition that collaborative intervention maximizes the teaching efforts of educators. Many of us have professionally prepared ourselves to build this bridge between our speech- language intervention and our students classroom instruction. Yet, often our initial collaborative efforts have left us in an uncomfortable zone as we navigated new and somewhat risky waters. CommunicationLab has helped me launch into, and successfully navigate through, this unfamiliar territory of collaboration, and I'm eager to share this model with you—my fellow colleagues.

The actual development of this collaborative program arose out of the work of two noteworthy professionals: Dr. Lena Rustin, manager of speech-language pathology in the Camden and Islington health districts in London, England, and author of *Social Skills and the Speech Impaired*, and Dr. Dick Mallard, Professor and Director of The Communications Disorders Program at southwest Texas State University. Lena and Dick are recognized nationally for their effective stuttering therapy model for children. Their approach involves the entire family by teaching all family members the social skills and speech techniques that will facilitate fluency and effective communication.

Working with Dick and Lena provided me with the insight and tools to approach ALL speech-language cases with a communication emphasis—that is, to offer all students an opportunity to learn communication skills that will support their improved speech, language, learning, and social functioning. I realized collaboration could begin at the core: COMMUNICATION! Communication skill training is a non-threatening, practical place to begin speech and language intervention since communication is so basic to everything else that we do in life. CommunicationLab was developed over a three-and-a-half-year period at Meadowbrook Elementary School in Northbrook, Illinois, and it continues to evolve.

CommunicationLab has produced such profound, positive effects on students' academic and social functioning that teachers have encouraged me to share the program by offering workshops to other professionals.

This book developed out of the incredibly supportive feedback I have received over the last five years from professionals around the country who strongly encouraged me to put this material into book form so they could implement CommunicationLab in their own schools. Initially, I hesitated to attempt capturing the program on paper since communication is more of a process than a product. Faced with continuing requests, I began work on the book. The results of these efforts, *CommunicationLab 1*, is a teaching manual that provides SLP's with all the elements they need to initiate their own collaborative programs, including the ability to tailor the Lab to their own professional styles and needs.

It's my sincere hope that the book I have created, *CommunicationLab 1*, will serve as a springboard to activate collaboration between SLP's and their students' classroom teachers, to provide support for direct speech-language services, and to add an in-class teaching component. Now the SLP can join efforts with the classroom teacher to teach their students communication skills that will support and encourage their academic and social success.

Dedication

To the teachers, parents, and students of Meadowbrook Elementary in Northbrook, Illinois. Because of their commitment to communication, CommunicationLab is now a reality for all children.

And to Warren Dodge for his inner commitment to this material and his belief in me every step of the way.

Acknowledgments

This book is the product of many years of communicating and collaborating with family, friends, teachers, parents, and students. I gratefully acknowledge many people for their contributions to the development of CommunicationLab, the collaborative program which has profoundly influenced my life and the children whom I have taught.

For the development and production of this book, I want to offer special thanks to the following people: Dr. Dick Mallard inspired me in graduate school to "challenge the system" and encouraged me not to let all the "yes buts" stop me from pursuing my ideas. I am equally grateful to Dick for the opportunity to work with him in his Summer Intensive Stuttering Program at Southwest Texas State University. This experience provided me with the original seeds for CommunicationLab.

Dr. Lena Rustin, author of *Social Skills and the Speech Impaired*, shared her social skills model involving families, encouraged me, and gave me inspiration for CommunicationLab.

Speech-language clinician and colleague Nancy Byrd shared her invaluable time and experiences in the early development stages of CommunicationLab. Without the collaborative, enthusiastic, committed efforts and contributions of the teachers and administrators at

Meadowbrook Elementary in Northbrook, Illinois (where CommunicationLab was first developed), CommunicationLab may have only remained a good idea.

Primary teachers Judy Pringle and Mary Stamos piloted the very first Labs in their classrooms. Their openness, insights, and natural communication gifts were instrumental in the Lab's ultimate success!

Meadowbrook Principal, Gerry Durcany, trusted my professional judgment and allowed me to provide speech and language services under a nontraditional model.

Dr. Jim Kucienski, Assistant Superintendent of Northbrook School District No. 28, supported and promoted my enthusiasm for the Lab.

Social Worker Betsy Tremulis helped me navigate the early development years of the Lab and made many insightful contributions.

Primary teacher Betty Moody and media specialist Jill Loomis contributed hours of labor to develop a video series of the Lab so parents could be involved in their children's educational programs.

Educational consultant Dr. Anita DeBoer initially encouraged me to share the Lab with fellow colleagues. I'm grateful for her continued support, encouragement, wisdom, and love as I continue with both my personal and professional growth.

The teaching staff at The Children's Health Council in Palo Alto, California, actively continue to refine this therapy model.

My parents, Ray and June, contributed excellent suggestions and expressed enthusiasm for my work.

To Beth and Bruce Kerr, Kittie Yohe, and Dianna Johansen for their expertise and commitment in creating the original CommunicationLab book.

I would like to offer special thanks to my loving husband and partner, Warren Dodge, for his belief and confidence in me and my vision for speech and language pathologists. His sense of humor, attentive listening, unconditional understanding, and reminders to trust my instincts encouraged me through the arduous writing process. Without his hours of brainstorming, challenge sessions, and motivational talks, this book may have been forever in the works.

Introduction

Communication is at the heart of the education process, albeit overlooked as the keystone to learning. His ability to master the components of communication is at the heart of a child's successful school experience.

Dr. Gilbert Herer, Presidential Address, 1989 ASHA Convention, St. Louis, Missouri

President Herer's insight into the connection between education and communication has given us the impetus to deliver speech and language services under a more comprehensive and functional umbrella. We no longer perceive of ourselves as solely SLP's, but rather as communication specialists ready to offer services that benefit ALL children and support their success in school. President Herer further supports this comprehensive shift by reminding us of the following:

> We SLP's and audiologists have a key role to play in meeting children's communication needs. We are a resource ready to make significant contributions to the communicative effectiveness of ALL school children, including those children with handicapping conditions. With our diagnostic and treatment abilities, we have a role to play in prevention and in early intervention with young children at-risk.

CommunicationLab is built on the connection between education and communication. The Lab is an effective collaborative program that will allow you, the SLP, to provide speech and language services under a meaningful and efficient framework. You no longer have to treat articulation, fluency, language, and voice disorders in isolation; instead you can work with the child as a whole person—A COMMUNICATOR—a message sender and receiver. In light of this perspective, you are faced with the following important questions:

- ◆ Can students get their messages across successfully?
- ◆ Do students have the skills to seek understanding?
- ◆ Do students know which classroom behaviors will encourage their peers and teachers to provide them with the help they need to be successful?
- ◆ Do students have the social skills and behaviors necessary to work in groups?
- ◆ Do students feel confident enough to risk academically and socially, so they can expand their knowledge and friendship base?
- ◆ What kind of problem-solving skills do students have to help them cope with the daily challenges of the classroom and of life?

With CommunicationLab, you and the classroom teacher can join together to provide your students with these essential classroom and life-survival skills. Once students have mastered these core communication skills, they'll have a sturdy framework to support their speech, language, academic, and social development. Furthermore, the Lab will provide the classroom teacher with classroom management tools that will promote a cooperative learning environment. Together, you and the classroom teacher can build a lasting professional relationship while providing effective, collaborative teaching for some of the most important people in your lives—your students!

Chapter 1
Principles of CommunicationLab

What is CommunicationLab?

CommunicationLab is a dramatic breakthrough in providing collaborative speech-language intervention to kindergarten through eighth-grade students in an interactive classroom-based program over a 10-week period. This highly effective and engaging program links the efforts of the speech-language pathologist (SLP), the classroom teacher, and the students' parents. You'll teach students the communication skills necessary for improving their academic and social functioning while facilitating the carryover of newly acquired speech and language skills from the therapy room to the classroom. The Lab is provided in conjunction with other direct clinical speech and language services.

Which grade levels are appropriate for this program?

The Lab is designed for students in kindergarten through eighth grade. This program is also effective with self-contained special education classrooms.

Each Lab suggests activities for younger and older students. *Younger students* refers to children in kindergarten through second grade, as well as self-contained classrooms. *Older students* refers to children in the third through eighth grades. If you have some classrooms that are more advanced or less sophisticated than others, use your own clinical judgment when determining which format is best for each class.

What can I do to adapt this program for my self-contained classrooms?

Since communication and social skills are typically the areas of greatest weakness for special education students, provide these classrooms with the Lab throughout the school year rather than just the customary 10 weeks. (If this isn't an option for you, 10 weeks is better than none.) By providing a year-round, 30-minute Lab for these classrooms, you can present the Lab at a pace that meets students' needs and gives them the repetition and reinforcement of each communication lesson that they typically require.

First present the Lab as directed, and then provide as many follow-up activities as necessary to support what was taught in the Lab. If a 30-minute session is too long a period for your students, present the Warm Up Activities on one day and the Role Plays on another. With the classroom teacher, determine when the students have grasped the communication concept, and then move on confidently to the next lesson. If a particular communication skill is difficult for your students to comprehend, you can repeat the lesson at another time during the school year. After presenting all of the concepts of CommunicationLab, address additional communication concerns that arise, like how to use leisure time, how to handle teasing, frustration, and disappointment. CommunicationLab 2[1] will give you additional lesson plans to build on students' communication knowledge following the initial 10-week program.

Who is involved in this collaboration?

You'll coordinate the collaboration among the classroom teacher, parents, and students. Throughout this book, I refer to you, the SLP, as the communication teacher, since I have found that this invites and maintains a non-threatening collaborative relationship. You may also find this useful as you begin to build collaborative teams in your own school.

Teacher Involvement

Since the classroom teacher is critical to the success of CommunicationLab, I recommend that you tune into each classroom teacher's needs and personal style, and ask her to work with you to tailor the CommunicationLab to her particular environment. The classroom teacher has all the information about the needs of her students, and therefore, is a key component in helping you create and implement a successful program.

When working with classroom teachers, view yourself as a contributing guest in the teacher's classroom. As a guest, listen, observe, and respect each teacher's professional style and emphasis in curriculum.

Teachers, like everyone else for that matter, have convictions about the best ways to educate children. For instance, one teacher may strive for a more academic environment, while the teacher next door values and seeks harmony and cooperation in his classroom. When entering a classroom, focus on communication since everyone agrees that good communication skills are necessary for successful learning. This approach will allow the classroom teacher to be the curriculum expert and you to be the communication specialist. Clear demarcation of roles makes for a non-threatening, cooperative relationship.

---

[1] Ellen Pritchard Dodge, *CommunicationLab 2*. LinguiSystems, Inc., East Moline, IL, 1994.

Learning Disabilities Teacher Involvement

Most likely, you and the learning disabilities teacher will have some of the same students on your caseloads, so uniting and consolidating your teaching efforts is practical and effective. CommunicationLab can be used as a vehicle to make this connection with the learning disabilities teacher.

First, determine which students you and the learning disabilities teacher have in common. Then, provide the teacher with these students' CommunicationLab schedules. Invite the teacher to observe her students participating in the Lab so she can become familiar with the vocabulary and techniques of the Lab.

Following this observation, have an informal meeting with the teacher to discuss each student's specific communication needs and to brainstorm some ideas for reinforcing improved communicative behavior. The learning disabilities teacher can provide you with additional insights about particular students' learning styles.

A second opportunity exists for the SLP and learning disabilities teacher to unite their teaching efforts. Following the 10-week CommunicationLab program, the learning disabilities teacher could conduct a complementary classroom-based program that not only targets students identified with special needs, but it also enhances the educational program for ALL students. For instance, a series on handwriting, memory, or organizational skills could be developed and provided during the same time period that CommunicationLab was presented.

Parent Involvement

Professionals in the field of speech-language pathology have long been aware of the need to incorporate parents and other family members into therapy to encourage the carryover of newly acquired speech and language skills. Faced with the reality of working parents, obtaining parental involvement can be an overwhelming and frustrating task. We continue to seek creative ways to communicate with parents so together we can provide children with a more comprehensive, effective educational program. CommunicationLab makes this important connection with parents in the following four ways.

◆ **Weekly letters to parents**

To provide parents with the background knowledge they need to support the school's efforts, send them an introductory letter before their child begins the Lab. Parents will also receive a weekly communication letter outlining what their child learned that week and providing suggestions for some interactive carryover activities for use at home.

Each week, photocopy the letter and give copies to the classroom teacher to send home with her students following the CommunicationLab lesson. If the classroom teacher is concerned about the students taking these letters home, mail them directly to the parents. Parents report that the weekly letters help them initiate conversations with their children and create a way for them to become involved in their children's educational program.

◆ **Parent Lab**

Suggested activities are provided in each lesson to actively involve parents in their child's communication development. Siblings should be encouraged to participate in the suggested activities.

◆ **Videotaping**

Videotaping can be used effectively to encourage parental involvement as illustrated by third grade-teacher, Betty Moody. Betty graciously volunteered to videotape the entire 10-week series in her class. She then created a video library so parents could check out the tapes to observe their child learning each week's communication lesson. To top it off, Betty convinced the local cable television network to carry the communication series.

This story illustrates how teachers can commit to CommunicationLab and make contributions that enrich and expand the program beyond what we could do on our own! Perhaps someone in your school or a parent could volunteer to videotape your CommunicationLab.

◆ **Parent review session**

Parents are invited to participate in the last session of CommunicationLab so they can see their children using all of their newly-refined communication skills. After the final session, you may decide to design and send home an evaluation form with the last parent letter, asking parents to provide you with feedback on how CommunicationLab worked for their children. You and the classroom teacher will feel deep satisfaction from all the supportive, positive comments offered by the parents.

Social Worker Involvement

Invite your school social worker to be a part of your collaborative team. Start by setting up a time to brainstorm how your two fields can complement each other when presenting CommunicationLab. Although it can add a new and exciting dimension to your classroom programming, including the school social worker isn't mandatory for the success of your program.

What skills are covered in CommunicationLab?

The communication curriculum focuses on the fundamental social skills that are involved in interacting with others, both socially and academically. While enhancing your students' communication skills, you'll notice an increase in their self-esteem and active learning behavior. Children become more receptive to processing, formulating, and learning when they're feeling good about themselves because they have more energy to spend on these processes. When they feel good about themselves, students are more willing to risk academically since making mistakes is less devastating.

This book will give you a springboard to launch your own CommunicationLab. As you read each lesson, note the additions and adjustments you want to make to customize the program. Classroom teachers will also have many valuable contributions.

CommunicationLab covers the following topics.

◆ What do good communicators do?

Brainstorm to discover the habits of good communicators.

◆ Observation

Read the situation before communicating so you can exercise good timing and appropriateness.

◆ Body Language

Observe nonverbal messages other people are sending and monitor your own non-verbal communication.

◆ Listening

Use the habits of active listeners, such as eye contact, head nods, and asking clarifying and verifying questions.

◆ Turn Taking

Enter and exit a conversation and/or activity appropriately, and include, rather than exclude, others.

◆ The Way We Communicate

Use your voice in a helpful, rather than hurtful, way, and self-correct when you catch yourself being hurtful.

◆ Praise

Give and receive praise.

◆ Criticism

Give and receive criticism in a way that encourages, rather than discourages, others' efforts.

◆ Success/Failure

Manage experiences of both success and failure by using techniques such as positive self-talk and flip the pancake.

◆ Parent Review

Parents attend the Lab to observe their children problem-solving and using good communication skills to create cooperation and harmony.

Why would I want to adopt this program for my school?

Demands on school-based SLP's are becoming increasingly unmanageable with escalating caseload sizes. SLP's have been challenging the traditional pull-out intervention programs as they learn about more effective and efficient ways to provide services to students with special needs. Many clinicians have turned to collaborative classroom-based models to create a more functional program. Unfortunately, they may experience resistance from teaching staff, administrators, and parents to this shift in service delivery. Many educators experience understandable anxiety about having to rede-

fine their roles in the educational system. Other clinicians want to move toward a collaborative classroom-based model but aren't sure how or where to begin. CommunicationLab will help you address both of these obstacles as you develop your own collaborative programming.

CommunicationLab will be one of the most meaningful, effective, and widely welcomed programs you'll implement in your school. The Lab is an effective vehicle to manage heavy caseloads. In addition, CommunicationLab is a non-threatening collaborative program that initiates collaboration at the core of education—COMMUNICATION! Research suggests that 70–80% of our waking life is spent communicating (Ward, J.R., 1990). But where in the curriculum is communication specifically taught? This void creates a significant opportunity for you to initiate a profound collaborative program and to provide children with skills they'll use throughout their lives.

What are the advantages of using this program?

◆ **Prevention and early intervention tool**

The Lab provides a preventive and early intervention tool since all students are in direct contact with you, and they are all taught skills that will encourage success in school.

◆ **Diagnostic tool**

The Lab will provide you with a diagnostic arena as you interact with students and teachers. When a teacher has a specific concern about a student, there's no need to set up an observation time since you'll be able to observe that student's speech and language skills during her next CommunicationLab.

◆ **Carryover tool**

The Lab will provide an opportunity for carryover intervention for the students on your caseload. During your regularly scheduled therapy time, you and your students can create signals to cue them to their speech and language objectives. Then while they're communicating in the Lab, your students can monitor their articulation, voice, language, and/or fluency under your supervision.

◆ Reduced stigma of special education

Providing the Lab on a school-wide basis will demystify special education as all students interact with and learn from you. Students on your speech-language caseload report that they feel less different because their peers have a positive impression of this special education service.

◆ Increased teaching time

Teachers will gain increased teaching time because students now have the communication tools to manage their own behaviors. When a teacher needs to intervene, he can use a common vocabulary. Teachers can just say a word or a phrase rather than having to speak in "chapters," as first grade teacher Judy Pringle puts it.

◆ Public relations benefits

As a side benefit, CommunicationLab will be a public relations bonanza! Since communication is universally valued, you can expect positive feedback from your teaching staff, students, administrators, and parents. Don't be surprised if surrounding school districts contact you to find out more about the Lab.

◆ Increased staff morale

Another benefit of CommunicationLab will be an overwhelming increase in staff morale. As you and the other adults involved in the program become more aware of your own communication skills, you'll notice less interrupting and better cooperation at building meetings. As students involved in the program become more aware of communication skills, they'll begin treating each other and adults with greater respect and consideration. This increase in positive school-wide communication will lead to students' improved academic and social functioning.

◆ Continued collaboration

CommunicationLab will be just the beginning of your meaningful collaboration with classroom teachers. Once you establish a professional relationship built on trust, respect, and a common purpose, continued collaboration with language and learning issues will be welcomed by the teaching staff. You'll strengthen your own professional confidence and teaching skills while managing a whole classroom. And, most importantly, students will develop the communication skills and classroom behaviors that will support learning.

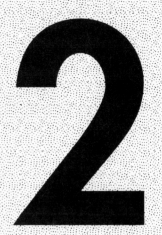

Chapter 2
Lab Organization

What is the format for each lesson?

Since communication is a process rather than a product, it was impossible to impose a single format upon each lesson for CommunicationLab. Although the lessons are similar, no two lessons have identical formats.

Springboard

The Lab will begin with a Springboard to activate your students' curiosity and previous knowledge about each communication skill. Springboards typically consist of a "captivating event" followed by stimulating questions and comments to ignite your students' interest. This question and commenting section will provide your students with an opportunity to brainstorm.

Occasionally, you or the classroom teacher will write your students' responses to the brainstorm on poster board or butcher paper. The classroom teacher can then refer to this list during the week when reinforcing the students' new communication skills. For instance, in the first lesson, *What Do Good Communicators Do?*, you and the classroom teacher will role-play poor communication skills so the students can discover the habits of good listeners. While you ask the questions, have the classroom teacher write down the students' responses.

What do good communicators do?

◆ use eye contact
◆ listen
◆ take turns
◆ use body language

15

Warm Up Activity

Each Lab includes Warm Up Activities that target that week's communication skill. Suggestions are provided for both younger and older students so you can design the Lab to meet each classroom's developmental needs.

Role Plays

The Role Play section is the heart of each Lab. Through role plays, your students will practice each skill and learn the consequences of good and poor communication. First, you and the classroom teacher will role play a problem or "poor communication" situation. Next, you'll debrief with your students to assess what happened because of poor communication. Then, students will have an opportunity to problem solve and role play again using "good communication." This process is described further in the *How is the role play section of the Lab organized?* section.

Wrap Up

In the Wrap Up section of the Lab, you'll provide your students with an opportunity to recap what they have learned about communication that day. The classroom teacher will help students think about how they might use these new communication skills in real life. The classroom teacher and students can brainstorm to develop a plan for how they will practice the new communication skill in the coming week. For instance, they may decide to create a nonverbal signal to remind interrupters to use better timing with their communication.

Communication Challenge

The communication challenge will provide a structured way for you to encourage students to practice the specific skills they learned that week. Each week, you'll review with your students to see if they were successful with the previous week's challenge or if they need more information in order to use the new communication skill.

Classroom Carryover Activities

Each Lab includes a "leave behind" activity sheet for the classroom teacher. The suggested activities will reinforce and extend the newly learned communication skills. Activities are designed so the classroom teacher can easily incorporate them into her day without much material or preparation time. You can also use these reinforcing activities with students on your caseload during their regular therapy sessions. Many of the suggested Carryover Activities are terrific for co-teaching a lesson with the classroom teacher. The *Monitor Turn Taking Activity* in Lesson 4 and the *Paraphrasing and Questioning Activity* in Lesson 5 are two good examples of lessons that "scream" for co-teaching.

How is the role play section of the Lab organized?
Suggested Role Plays

Each role play is designed to target communication skills necessary for school, peer relations, and home. Each lesson will provide you with suggested role plays to target these crucial areas. Many SLP's find that the role plays provided in the Lab can be taught throughout the year, rather than in 10 weeks. Choose one role play or as many as are needed for your students to grasp each communication concept. These suggested role plays have come from classroom teachers' observations and represent many of the communication problems that are barriers to learning and positive social interactions. You and the classroom teacher will have many role-play ideas of your own. You will design role plays during your pre-collaboration meeting with the teacher. (See *Pre-Lab Meeting* on page 33.)

Assessing Role Plays

Following each role play, call "freeze!" Then, provide your students with an opportunity to talk about what they observed. The suggested brainstorming questions will help your students discover the following:

◆ Who wasn't a good communicator?

◆ Which communication skill wasn't used?

◆ What could the students have done differently to make the situation better?

This section of the Lab will increase your students' abilities to think of all the options that are available to them when responding in any situation. Be careful not to debrief too much as students will lose interest. They usually enjoy the action of role playing more.

Problem Solving

After assessing the role plays, your students will be ready to role play the situation again using improved communication. For instance, if in the first role play, a student interrupted the teacher, now the student could communicate with better timing by waiting his turn. This portion of the Lab will provide your students with an opportunity to compare and contrast their use of good and poor communicative behavior. This experience will enable your students to be better problem solvers when challenged with communication problems.

How can I help my younger and special education students participate in role playing?

For younger students and students with special needs, initially role play poor communication behavior for the students to identify. Next, give these students an opportunity to role play a situation again using improved communication. Many classes will need a little help to participate in these re-role plays, and if a particular class is floundering, you may wish to narrate how to use improved communication. When narrating, you simply say exactly what you want the students to do. For example, you might say, "Then Caitlin waited for Ms. Owens to finish correcting the math papers so she could ask the teacher for help with her reading."

How do older students handle role playing?

You'll find that your older students will love role playing and will turn into real hams in front of their peers. In fact, after about four CommunicationLabs, you and the classroom teacher will no longer have to participate in the role plays since your students will love to role play both the right and wrong way to communicate. In addition, your students will want to begin developing the role plays on their own. This is ideal. Your students will problem solve some of their own real-life situations that make learning and friendships difficult. Older students also benefit from designing role plays in small groups and then performing in front of the class.

When this happens, your role will become that of the facilitator who asks the right questions to help your students come up with the appropriate role plays. Suggestions for facilitating the development of these role plays are included in each lesson. Following your students' role plays, use the provided assessment questions (outlined for younger students) to help your students discuss the consequences of using good and poor communication habits.

What is the role of the teachers during the role plays?

The role-playing section of the Lab tends to be the highlight for both your students and the classroom teacher. Teachers will feel great relief when they get to imitate classroom behaviors that get on their nerves, like constant interruptions, telling on another student, whining, and poor attention. Additionally, you and the classroom teacher will win your students' hearts as you play the part of "poor communicators." Students get a kick out of seeing their teachers out of character and acting silly.

As you and the classroom teacher design role plays, give the classroom teacher the funniest and most exciting roles. The teacher who isn't role playing can serve as the facilitator who asks the assessment questions provided in each lesson. If the classroom teacher isn't comfortable role playing, she can just observe as students will love to role play with you.

Are there any additional components of the Lab?

Vocabulary

Yes, the vocabulary is the driving force behind CommunicationLab and an extremely important feature of this collaborative program. Teachers and parents report that the vocabulary makes it easy to communicate with the children since everyone "speaks the same language." Prior to your first lesson with your students, provide both the classroom teacher and parents with the *CommunicationLab Vocabulary* handout (Chapter 4, page 34).

Throughout the program, you'll model how to use the vocabulary to facilitate improved communication. Whenever it's appropriate, you'll comment on communication by using the

vocabulary from the program. For instance, you might say, "Terrific Bruce, you *observed* that I was busy, and you didn't interrupt," or "You remembered to use *thinking time.*"

Soon students, teachers, and parents will begin using the vocabulary. An example of this comes from a true story about a second-grade girl and boy. Picture a typical boy chasing a girl while the girl warns, "Don't chase me. Don't chase me." Interestingly, this scene is somewhat different from most chase scenes since this young boy was equipped with the communication skills and vocabulary of the program as illustrated by his reply, "You're sending me a mixed message. Your words are saying, 'Don't chase me,' but your body language is saying, 'Chase me.'" I'd say that was pretty clear communication!

Materials

Very few materials are necessary to conduct this program. Props for role plays you create can be found right in the classroom. For example, you may use desks, chalkboard, text books, scissors, glue, and other school supplies that are on hand. When designing role plays, you can be elaborate or simple.

Teachable Moments

Predictable communication problems will occur while teaching the Lab. This is your "teachable moment"[2] to prompt improved communication. For example, when Tim changes the subject, you can prompt, "Tim, do you want to change the subject? You can ask me."

Teachable moments are not part of your lesson plan, but they often have a positive impact on communication in the classroom.

---

[2] Ellen Pritchard Dodge, *Teachable Moments for Classroom Communication.* LinguiSystems, Inc., East Moline, IL, 1994.

Tips for Using This Book

Use the *Lesson Plan Worksheet* (Chapter 4, page 39) to help you prepare for each communication lesson. After reading each chapter, note the important points on the worksheet, put it on a clipboard, and bring it to class. Use the Personal Notes section to summarize how the session went. You might include notes about students you need to target, as well as other observations you make about a specific class. You may also wish to make notes about what adjustments or additions you'd like to make the next time you teach this class.

Chapter 3
Scheduling and Preparation

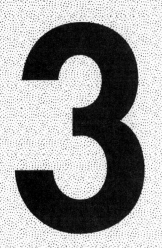

How do I begin?

Offer an informal, 20-minute in-service presentation that creates curiosity, enthusiasm, and interest in the Lab. This in-service can be handled in one of two ways, based on your professional style and needs.

The first approach comes from educational consultant Dr. Anita DeBoer. Rather than telling your staff why they should want a program such as CommunicationLab, conduct a mini needs assessment. This will heighten teachers' awareness of communication and create an internal need for the Lab. Begin this in-service with a general overview of the Lab, and then conduct the needs assessment using the *Needs Assessment* (Chapter 4, page 30).

Another approach for this mini in-service is to provide your staff with a brief overview of CommunicationLab, including how it will be useful to them as classroom teachers. Tailor the *In-Service Outline* (Chapter 4, page 29) to your staff's particular needs and styles.

Regardless of which approach you take for this in-service, remember to ask yourself, "What's in it for the teacher?" As you are well aware, teachers have incredible demands placed on their time, and they are understandably hesitant to add one more thing to their busy schedules. However, once teachers become aware of how useful this program can be for them, you'll increase your chances of getting volunteers to pilot CommunicationLab with you.

Your goal for this in-service is to find one teacher who is willing to incorporate this novel program into her schedule. Chances are that once the Lab gets off the ground in one classroom, the program will sell itself based on the positive results the first volunteer experiences. After conducting the first Lab, you'll have an "inside coach" who will encourage other teachers to get involved. Other teachers will soon be asking you when you can schedule their classes for CommunicationLab. Gradually, CommunicationLab will be incorporated into more and more classrooms. This natural progression of the Lab will allow you time to gain confidence and additional experience in directing it.

As with any program, a few procedures must precede the teachers' actual participation in CommunicationLab. These include tasks such as in-servicing, scheduling, and planning. Use the *CommunicationLab Checklist* (Chapter 4, page 28) to keep track of each procedure as it's completed before you kick off your first lesson on communication.

How do I schedule teachers for the Lab?

One of the first things SLP's say to me when they learn about this program is, "This sounds great, but where do you find time?" My answer is always the same:

> "I can't afford not to create time for the Lab. The Lab is the core of my therapy (because it supports my direct therapy) and is my own personal sanity saver. Results of the Lab are so rewarding, it saves me from feeling burned out. Students throughout the school greet me in the hall and are eager to tell me anecdotes about how they're using the skills from the Lab. Other teachers also value the Lab, as indicated by special education teacher Denise Foss who reports, 'The Lab is ten times more effective than any pull-out program.' In addition, teaching in isolation can be lonely and monotonous. Interacting with different classroom teachers adds variety, humor, and creativity to the day. So, CommunicationLab is my first priority."

Revolving Schedule

CommunicationLab is extremely manageable and effective when offered to classroom teachers on a revolving schedule. Limit the Lab to five classrooms at a time so you can continue to provide students with direct therapy services as well. When the first five classrooms complete the program, offer the Lab to the next five classrooms on your waiting list. To set up this revolving schedule, proceed as follows:

◆ At the beginning of the school year, block out five 30-minute sessions on your schedule for CommunicationLab sessions.

◆ Choose different days of the week and different times of the day so you can accommodate all the teachers' teaching schedules. For example, you might schedule one session on Monday from 9:00 to 9:30 a.m. and another on Tuesday from 1:00 to 1:30 p.m.

◆ Be sure to check your school calendar to accommodate the many holidays throughout the year.

◆ Plan CommunicationLab when students on your caseload are scheduled for pull-out therapy. Following the 10-week program, students can return to their pull-out sessions. The 10 weeks spent in the classroom will not only help to create an improved learning environment, but it will give you an arena to coach your speech and language students to use their new speech and language skills in the classroom.

Notification of Lab Availability

Following your schoolwide in-service presentation, determine the days and times you'll be offering CommunicationLab, fill out *CommunicationLab Sign-Up Sheet,* (Chapter 4, page 31), make copies, and send to the classroom teachers.

On the handouts, the teachers will indicate their first, second, and third choices for when they would like their class to participate in the Lab. After you receive the completed handouts, schedule the classes on your revolving schedule. For example, you can schedule Mr. Shepp's class the first 10 weeks at a specific time, and then use that same time slot for Ms. Downey's class when Mr. Shepp's Lab is over.

It's your clinical choice as to which classrooms receive the Lab first. Make sure the kindergartners are among the first students since they'll be new to the building, and the Lab will immediately set the tone and establish the rules for their new school.

Scheduling Form

After you plan your schedule for CommunicationLab, notify classroom teachers by completing and distributing *CommunicationLab Schedule* (Chapter 4, page 32). Include the day of the week, time of day, and dates when their class is scheduled for the Lab.

Keep in mind that this is a new program for you as well, so be careful in your enthusiasm not to schedule too many classrooms at once. It's better to start with one classroom and get your feet wet than to become overwhelmed by taking on too many classes at once and then having to quit because the caseload is unmanageable. Allow yourself extra planning and thinking time during your first run through the program. Start with a class with which you're already comfortable. Once you have some success under your belt, begin adding one or two additional classes. Before you know it, your entire school will have an opportunity to participate in the Lab.

Pre-Collaboration Meeting

After you schedule all of the classrooms for this year's CommunicationLab, plan a 45-minute pre-Lab meeting with each participating classroom teacher. Co-design the Lab to meet their specific students' needs. Perhaps you are thinking, "Just what I need, another meeting!" This reaction is understandable since every SLP knows that one sure saboteur of collaboration is all of the extra meetings and all of the planning time that is required. Good news! This pre-Lab meeting will be your only scheduled meeting. Use it to plan, organize, and connect with the classroom teacher before you join forces to create a cooperative communicative classroom! There are some educators who create time to meet on a weekly basis to co-plan their Lab lessons. If this works for you, great!

Prior to the pre-Lab meeting, read the Introduction section of each communication lesson to familiarize yourself with the skills that you and the classroom teacher will be targeting during each Lab. A quick review of the Creating Role Plays section for each Lab will give you additional help designing role plays with the classroom teachers.

What are the goals of the pre-Lab meeting?

◆ Review the *CommunicationLab Schedule* so you and the classroom teacher can begin to focus on the skills on which your students will be working.

◆ Provide the teacher with the *CommunicationLab Vocabulary* handout (Chapter 4, page 34) so you can share a common vocabulary that targets improved communication.

◆ Identify the students' communication strengths and weaknesses.

23

- Co-design role plays with the classroom teacher.
- Clarify what each of you will do when presenting CommunicationLab.

Each of these five objectives are discussed in more detail below.

CommunicationLab Schedule

Begin the pre-Lab meeting by reviewing *CommunicationLab Schedule*. Briefly summarize why each communication skill is important to learning.

Vocabulary

As stated earlier, the vocabulary of the program is an essential component of CommunicationLab. Provide the classroom teacher with the *CommunicationLab Vocabulary* handout. Ask the teacher if she has any additional vocabulary or phrases that she already uses with her class. Chances are that each teacher has already established some effective vocabulary and methods to manage his classroom. For instance, social worker Betsy Tremulis reminds students as they board the school bus, "Hands and feet to self," while primary teacher Mary Stamos reminds her students to "L and L" which is to look and listen.

After you and the classroom teacher share your vocabularies, you can both "speak the same language," which will help create a consistent and cooperative learning environment.

Tailoring the Lab

As you go over each area of CommunicationLab, explain that you'd like the classroom teacher to indicate the strengths and weaknesses of her students in regards to each skill. As the teacher shares her concerns and insights about her students' communicative behavior, take notes on

the *Co-Designing Role Plays* handout (Chapter 4, page 36). These notes will help you create role plays that will go to the heart of the students' communication difficulties.

To help you direct this conversation, use the facilitative questions following each communication skill. Encourage the teacher to give you the names of specific students she would like to target during each Lab. This way, when it comes time for role playing, you'll know which students will benefit from being involved. For example, if Lisa always interrupts, then she may need to experience what it feels like to be interrupted.

Co-Designing Role Plays

After the classroom teacher shares her concerns and insights about her students' communicative behaviors, you'll be ready to co-design one role play for each communication topic. For instance, for *The Way We Communicate* lesson, if the teacher describes students who use a demanding or whining tone of voice when asking for help, you might design a role play where the teacher plays the part of a whining student, and a student plays the role of the teacher. This way, students will learn the consequences of communicating with a whining or demanding tone of voice. They'll then have an opportunity to problem solve more effective ways to communicate.

After you and the classroom teacher design a role play for each lesson, create additional role plays from your own observations. Suggestions for additional role plays are provided for each lesson. Occasionally role plays may turn out differently than you expected because students may say and/or do something differently than instructed. On these occasions, simply discuss the outcome as it relates to communication.

Arrive at the classroom five minutes before the scheduled Lab time so you and the classroom teacher can go over the day's activities. Reassure the teacher that the Lab isn't a Broadway production, but an informal program. You'll have an opportunity to talk between role plays to clarify who is going to do what.

Clarifying Roles

It's important that both you and the classroom teacher feel like equal contributing partners in this collaborative effort. To help create this relationship, it's helpful if each of you know what your role will be when presenting the Lab. To conclude the pre-Lab meeting, select a lesson from this book and outline the format of the Lab by explaining what happens in the Springboard, Warm Up, Role Playing, Wrap Up, and Communication Challenge sections. Further explain that you'll bring a clipboard with an outline of the sequence of events for each day. Reassure the classroom teacher that the Lab is a process, not a product. There is no right or wrong way to conduct the program.

How do you document progress?

Accountability is an essential component of all intervention efforts. You'll want to collect data to support the positive changes that occur as a result of the Lab. Use both subjective and objective data when evaluating students' progress.

You might want to use the *CommunicationLab Profile*[3] to assess your students' progress pre- and post-Lab. This informal assessment will give you an overall profile of communication competence.

◆ Subjective Evaluation

Prior to conducting CommunicationLab, get parents' and teachers' observations about students' communicative behaviors. Specifically, ask parents and adults to observe and comment on students' competencies in each of the communication areas covered in the Lab.

- ◆ How do students get in and out of conversations?
- ◆ Do they frequently interrupt?
- ◆ Do students read the nonverbal cues in their environment?
- ◆ What kind of listening behaviors do they have?

Record the teachers' and parents' observations along with your own clinical observations of the students' communicative behaviors. At the end of the 10-week program, obtain a second report from these sources to note any positive communication changes that have occurred.

◆ Objective Evaluation

It's equally important to obtain objective data for documentation. This can be easily obtained by gathering baseline information on a particular communication skill prior to a student's participation in the Lab. For instance, if you're targeting turn-taking behavior, note the average number of interruptions a student makes in a given subject area. This baseline information can be obtained by you or by the classroom teacher.

Ask the classroom teacher to select a subject area such as reading, and then count the number of a student's interruptions over a five-day period. Calculate the average number of interruptions for this student.

After the Lab, compare the students' previous average number of interruptions to her subse-

---

[3] Ellen Pritchard Dodge, *CommunicationLab Profile*. LinguiSystems, Inc., East Moline, IL, 1994.

quent number of interruptions. The classroom teacher could easily solicit a student volunteer to keep track of a student's turn-taking behavior. When done in game form, like a T.V. survey, students will enjoy collecting data for teachers.

The combination of both this qualitative and quantitative data will provide you with the support you'll need for future collaborative teaching efforts.

What do I do after this 10-week program?

CommunicationLab works on a revolving schedule, so when one classroom is finished with the program, you can offer the Lab to the next class on the waiting list. Typically, by spring, you'll have provided the Lab to all the classrooms in your school. The following school year you can offer the introductory CommunicationLab to kindergartners and a follow-up CommunicationLab for the rest of the grade levels. Begin the follow-up program with a brainstorm.

- ◆ What do we remember about good communication?
- ◆ Which communication skills is our class good at?
- ◆ Which communication skills does our class need to work on?

From the information your students provide during this initial meeting, you and the classroom teacher will design the follow-up Labs. Following are some suggestions:

- ◆ How do you play in a threesome?
- ◆ What makes a game go well?
- ◆ What makes a conversation go well?
- ◆ How can we handle frustration?

The success you experience with *Communication-Lab 1* will naturally prepare you for a follow-up program the next year. *CommunicationLab 2* provides you with information and additional lessons to continue the Lab.

Continued Collaboration

By late spring, when all classrooms have participated in the Lab, you'll find yourself with some available 30-minute openings in your schedule. (A miracle, right?) I have used these openings for two purposes. First, I typically find the spring to be a heavy referral season, so now I have time in my schedule for those additional diagnostics and end-of-the-year meetings. It used to be that I had to cancel scheduled therapy sessions so I could attend to all the incoming referrals and meetings. Talk about stress and sabotaging relationships with classroom teachers! With these 30-minute openings, I rarely have to cancel scheduled sessions with students.

These 30-minute openings also provide me with an another opportunity to collaborate with classroom teachers in the content areas of the curriculum. Now that we have developed a working professional relationship, and students have improved communicative behavior, we're prepared to collaborate on language and learning issues. This partnership has been an extremely effective and efficient way to provide speech and language services to the numerous students on my caseload. You can expect similar success as you begin or continue your collaboration with the three essential partners: the classroom teacher, the student, and the parent.

Chapter 4
Handouts for
CommunicationLab

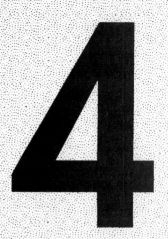

You will use the following handouts to get CommunicationLab off the ground in your school:

◆ CommunicationLab Checklist

◆ In-Service Outline

◆ Needs Assessment/Rating Scale for the Needs Assessment

◆ CommunicationLab Sign-Up Sheet

◆ CommunicationLab Schedule

◆ Pre-Lab Meeting Sign-Up Sheet/Notice of pre-Lab Meeting

◆ CommunicationLab Vocabulary

◆ Co-Designing Role Plays Worksheet

◆ Lesson Plan Worksheet

◆ Introductory Letter to Parents

Make photocopies of these forms for each CommunicationLab.

CommunicationLab Checklist

Use this checklist to keep track of your CommunicationLab scheduling.

_____ Provide a schoolwide in-service, using the *In-Service Outline* or *Needs Assessment/ Rating Scale for the Needs Assessment.*

_____ Determine the days and times you'll offer the Lab. Add this schedule to *CommunicationLab Sign-Up Sheet.*

_____ Send teachers the completed *CommunicationLab Sign-Up Sheet.*

_____ Schedule classes for the Lab using the *CommunicationLab Schedule.*

_____ Send teachers the completed *CommunicationLab Schedule.*

_____ Send teachers the *Pre-Lab Meeting Sign-Up Sheet/Notice of pre-Lab Meeting.*

_____ Schedule teachers for the pre-Lab meeting and provide them with written notice by returning the *Notice of pre-Lab Meeting.*

During the 45-minute pre-Lab meeting, do the following:

_____ Review the *CommunicationLab Schedule* and the *CommunicationLab Vocabulary* handout with the teacher.

_____ Create role plays with the *Co-Designing Role Plays Worksheet.*

Following the pre-Lab meeting, do the following:

_____ Send parents the introductory letter and the *CommunicationLab Vocabulary* handout.

_____ Prior to presenting each lesson, fill out the *Lesson Plan Worksheet.*

_____ Conduct Lessons 1-9 of CommunicationLab.

_____ Conduct Lesson 10 — the parent review session!

In-Service Outline

Introduction (5 minutes)

◆ Present a brief summary of the traditional role of the SLP.

◆ Briefly explain how SLP's no longer need to treat articulation, language, fluency, and voice in isolation, but they can look at a child as a whole person: a communicator, a message sender, and a receiver.

Specifics of CommunicationLab (15 minutes)

(See Chapter 2 for details.)

◆ What is CommunicationLab?

◆ Which skills are covered in the Lab?

◆ How long is the program?

◆ Who is involved in the Lab?

◆ Why would I want to have the Lab in my classroom?

◆ What is the format of the Lab?

◆ How can I sign up for the Lab?

Question and Answer Period (5 minutes)

Needs Assessment

Following a brief description of Communication-Lab, tell the classroom teachers that you'd like to do a quick needs assessment to see if there is a need for this type of program in their classrooms.

Provide teachers with a sheet of paper and ask them to respond *yes* or *no* to questions you read aloud. Then, help the teachers score their results by using the *Rating Scale for the Needs Assessment*.

Wrap up this in-service by briefly explaining how CommunicationLab can address some of the teachers' concerns about their students' communicative behaviors.

1. Do you have students in your class who come to your desk to get help when you are in the middle of helping another student?

2. Do you find that you have to repeat directions because students failed to listen the first time?

3. Are you constantly reminding students to raise their hands before they speak?

4. Do you have some students who rarely get included in group activities?

5. Do you find that some of your students need to be reminded to turn around and face the front of the room?

6. Do you have students who have to be first in everything?

7. Are you tired of having to play the part of the referee when your students get into arguments?

8. Are you concerned about a student's self-esteem because you overhear him refer to himself as "dummy" or because he says things to himself like, "I can't do anything right"?

9. Does it feel like "pulling teeth" to get some students to contribute to class discussions?

10. Do you have students who make fun of others' mistakes or shortcomings?

Rating Scale for the Needs Assessment

Ask your teachers to total their *yes/no* responses and then listen as you read the following ratings.

♦ If you answered *yes* to 6 out of 10 questions, you're saying that your class has a mild need for CommunicationLab. I'd like to tell you more about the program.

♦ If you answered *yes* to 7 out of 10 questions, you're saying that your class has a moderate need for CommunicationLab. When can we get together and talk?

♦ If you answered *yes* to 8 out of 10 questions, you're saying that your class has a severe need for CommunicationLab. When can we start the Lab?

♦ If you answered *yes* to 9 out of 10 questions, you're saying your class has a profound need for CommunicationLab. Can we start the Lab tomorrow?

♦ If you answered *yes* to 10 out of 10 questions, you're saying that your class is suffering from a massive communication breakdown. Can we start the Lab today?

CommunicationLab Sign-Up Sheet

Thank you for attending the CommunicationLab In-Service. I'm looking forward to getting this exciting program off the ground in many classrooms. Please fill out and return this form so I can begin scheduling classes to participate in this dynamic 10-week series.

I appreciate your enthusiasm and support for building our children's communication skills since communication is basic to everything that your students will do throughout their lives!

Name _____

_____ Yes, please include me in this year's CommunicationLab.

_____ No, we're unable to include this program in our schedule this year.

_____ I don't have enough information about CommunicationLab. Could we meet for ten minutes to discuss this program further?

Following are the days and times the Lab will be offered this year. Please indicate your preference by selecting your first, second, and third choice. As soon as I have your class scheduled, I'll let you know your starting date.

CommunicationLab Schedule

Your class has been scheduled for CommunicationLab as follows:

Lab Lesson	Day	Dates	Time
1			
2			
3			
4			
5			
6			
7			
8			
9			
10			

Pre-Lab Meeting Sign-Up Sheet

Now that your class is scheduled for CommunicationLab, I'd like to schedule a 45-minute meeting with you so we can tailor the Lab to meet your students' needs. Please provide me with three options for days and times you are free to meet with me to co-plan your Lab.

	Day	Time
1		
2		
3		

- -

Notice of pre-Lab Meeting

I have scheduled our pre-Lab meeting for _____ at _____.

See you then!

CommunicationLab Vocabulary

Observation
It's important to assess the situation before we begin to communicate so we can communicate appropriately and with good timing. Remind students to ask themselves, "Is the person I want to talk to busy or talking to someone else?"

Body Language
We use our entire body when sending and receiving messages. Our facial expressions and body gestures send messages along with our words. Help students observe body language to give them more information about the message. Remind students to ask themselves, "What is the speaker feeling? What message is my face and body sending?"

Mixed Messages
Sometimes our words and body language don't match. Our words say one thing, and our body language says another. For instance, your words may say you aren't mad, but your body language communicates that you're still upset. Help students send CLEAR messages with matching words and body language.

Listening
Following are habits we can observe in a good listener:

◆ Eye contact: Look at the person with whom you are communicating.

◆ Head nods: Move your head up and down to show you're following the speaker.

◆ Listening noises: Let the speaker know you're listening by using an occasional "Oh, Umm," or "Wow."

◆ Comment and Question: Comment on and ask questions about the subject so the speaker is aware of your interest.

Talking About Talking
There are often times we can't give someone our full attention while listening because we're doing something else. By talking about talking we can let the speaker know that we're listening, but that we also need to continue doing what we're doing. For instance, if you are cooking when your child starts a conversation, you could say, "I'm listening, but I need to continue stirring so the chili doesn't burn."

Turn Taking
Students need to be reminded to use their observation skills to enter and exit conversations without interrupting. Remind students to ask themselves, "Am I talking too much?" or "Do I need to contribute more to the conversation?"

Self-Correct	We can **catch and correct** ourselves when we make mistakes. For instance, if we accidentally interrupt, we can say, "Excuse me." If we use an unkind tone of voice, we can apologize and say it again in a nicer way.
Thinking Time	Help students take the time to think about a situation rather than just react to it. Remind students to ask themselves, "How can I best handle this situation?" Encourage students to use thinking time for learning and speaking purposes. Often students need additional time to process information before they're ready to respond. Therefore, encourage them to say, "May I have some thinking time?"
The Way	The *way* we communicate, or our tone of voice and body language, can change the meaning of a message. When students use a polite tone of voice, praise them for communicating in a considerate way. Likewise, when students forget and use a hurtful, demanding, or whining tone of voice, remind them to communicate in a way that is more positive.
Self-Talk	Whether or not we realize it, we all have an ongoing internal dialogue with ourselves. This dialogue can either be encouraging or discouraging to us. For instance, when you observe a child make a mistake, do you hear her say things like, "I can't do anything right?" If so, we can help our students by modeling positive self-talk by saying encouraging things to ourselves like, "I'm going to get it right this time."

Co-Designing Role Plays Worksheet

Use the following questions to initiate a discussion about each communication topic with the classroom teacher. Encourage the teacher to "paint a picture" of what her students' communication behavior looks like so together you can design appropriate role plays.

Classroom Teacher _____

Observation

◆ Do your students ever fail to observe before they communicate. For example, do they ask for help when you're busy helping another student?

◆ What else do you wish your students would be more observant of in the classroom? On the playground?

Observation Role Plays	Target Students

Body Language

What negative, nonverbal messages do students send in your classroom or on the playground? For instance, do students roll their eyes or yawn when you're teaching, or do they give their peers dirty looks?

Body Language Role Plays	Target Students

Listening

◆ Tell me about your students' listening skills.

◆ When do your students experience the most difficulty listening?

Listening Role Plays	Target Students

Turn Taking

◆ Do you have students who constantly interrupt? Tell me about these interruptions.

◆ Do you have students who rarely contribute to class discussions? Tell me about them.

◆ Do you have students who are constantly excluded from group play? What does this look like?

Turn Taking Role Plays	Target Students

The Way We Communicate

◆ Tell me about the tones of voice students use while communicating with each other and with you. For instance, do your students ever use a whining or demanding tone of voice? When?

Way Role Plays	Target Students

Praise

◆ Do your students give each other praise very often?

◆ When could they praise each other more?

◆ How do your students react when they receive praise? For instance, do any of your students get embarrassed or reject the praise?

Praise Role Plays	Target Students

Criticism

◆ Do you observe your students putting each other down through teasing or criticism? What does this look like?

Criticism Role Plays	Target Students

Success/Failure

◆ How do your students handle success? Do you observe boasting?

◆ How do your students handle failure? Do you have students who grow discouraged and quit, or talk negatively about themselves? Tell me about it.

Success/Failure Role Plays	Target Students

Lesson Plan Worksheet

Classroom teacher _____

Communication topic _____

Springboard
Warm Up
School Role Plays
Friendship Role Plays
Home Role Plays
Wrap Up
Communication Challenge
Personal Notes (use reverse side)

Dear Parents,

Communication is at the core of learning and developing self-esteem. We're pleased to tell you that our class will be participating in a 10-week program to improve students' communication skills. The program is called CommunicationLab and will be taught by me, the school's speech-language pathologist, and by your child's classroom teacher.

The Lab will meet once a week to cover the following topics:

- What do good communicators do?
- Observation
- Body Language
- Listening
- Turn Taking
- The Way We Communicate
- Praise
- Criticism
- Success and Failure

We'll also have a Parent's Day at the end of the 10 weeks so students can share what they've learned about communication.

To increase the effectiveness of this program, we'd like to coordinate our efforts with yours at home. Each week, you'll receive a letter that describes the communication skill we'll be practicing. These weekly letters will provide useful tips on how you can encourage your child's improved communication. They're also good conversation starters for you and your child.

In addition, we'll provide you with the vocabulary of Communication-Lab, since using the "same language" at home and at school will help students be more successful at acquiring these new skills.

We encourage you to share your concerns and insights about communication with us so we can provide a meaningful communication experience for your child.

We look forward to working with you to help your child develop one of life's most important skills—COMMUNICATION!

Sincerely,

Chapter 5
CommunicationLab Lessons

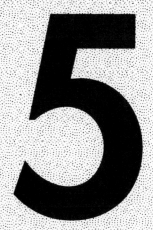

This chapter has nine lessons to teach communication skills to your students. Customize the lessons to meet the needs of each classroom. The tenth lesson is a Parent Review where parents can observe their children demonstrating the communication skills they've learned.

Lesson 1 introduces your students to the habits of what good communicators do.

Lesson 2 helps students learn how to read a situation before communicating to encourage good timing.

Lesson 3 moves your students beyond words to observe nonverbal messages and body language.

Lesson 4 teaches your students the importance of being good listeners.

Lesson 5 helps your students improve their turn-taking skills.

Lesson 6 focuses your students' attention on the way they communicate rather than on what they're saying.

Lesson 7 offers students ways to send and receive praise.

Lesson 8 demonstrates how students can send and receive constructive criticism.

Lesson 9 teaches students how to communicate with themselves and with others when experiencing successes and failures.

Lesson 10 is the Parent Review.

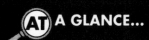

A GLANCE...

This chapter includes nine Lab lessons to help your students:

◆ learn what good communicators do

◆ improve their observation skills

◆ understand what body language is

◆ learn the importance of being good listeners

◆ improve their turn-taking skills

◆ focus on the way they communicate, rather than on what they're saying

◆ send and receive praise

◆ send and receive constructive criticism

◆ learn how to accept successes and failures

The tenth lesson will give your students a chance to demonstrate their improved communication skills to their parents.

Lesson 1: What Do Good Communicators Do?

You're about to introduce your students to the unspoken curriculum in school and in life. That is, you'll be teaching them the rules, communication, and behaviors that will enable them to learn and live more harmoniously with others. These life skills that you and the classroom teacher will teach your students may be the most important tools they'll acquire throughout their academic careers.

You're also beginning your collaboration with teachers at the core, COMMUNICATION. This non-threatening, meaningful beginning will serve as a springboard to future significant collaborations.

Vocabulary

eye contact: looking at each other's eyes while communicating

body language: communicating nonverbal messages using facial expressions and body gestures

observation: looking at the situation before communicating so one can communicate appropriately with good timing

listening: seeking understanding while using the habits of a good listener, such as eye contact, head nods, making listening noises, and commenting and questioning on the subject

turn taking: entering and exiting a conversation with good timing

the Way: using tone of voice and body language to change the meaning of the message

praise: expressing approval for, or admiration of, another's efforts

criticism: evaluating or judging another's efforts

success/failure: communicating to one's self and others when experiencing success and failure

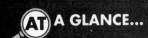

AT A GLANCE...

In this communication lesson, you'll be teaching your students how to:

◆ use brainstorming to become more flexible problem solvers

◆ become aware of the skills good communicators use

◆ discover reasons to improve their communication so they can improve their school and home functioning and peer relations

stay on the subject: contributing to a conversation on the subject

normal volume: using a speaking voice that isn't too loud or soft

clear speech: enunciating while speaking

normal rate of speech: speaking at an appropriate speed

adequate distance: allowing an adequate space between communicators

don't fidget: avoiding distracting a speaker or listener with restless movements

Materials

small, soft ball

poster board labeled "What Do Good Communicators Do?"

any props needed for the role plays you create

Springboard

To get this novel program off the ground, have the classroom teacher welcome you. Her enthusiasm will be contagious and will motivate the entire group to participate.

Greet the students and acknowledge the students from your caseload. Comment on how many of the students are already familiar to you because you're their speech and language teacher. Extend your role by explaining that you're also a communication teacher. Ask to see who can tell you what communication is.

Warm Up

Sending and Receiving Messages

Help your students understand that communication consists of sending and receiving messages. Equate communication to a ball game. Toss the ball to a student who looks prepared

to catch, and explain that it takes one person to throw the ball and another person to catch it. Just like in communication, you need a sender and a receiver.

◆ Communication Received

Ask the student to pass the ball back to you. Fail to catch it. Ask your students what happened. They'll talk about your missing the ball, which will allow you to explain that, like a ball game, when we talk, sometimes people don't listen to catch our message.

◆ Communication Missed

Next, toss the ball to another student so it barely reaches him. Again, explore with your students what happened. Explain that messages have to be sent loud enough for people to receive them.

◆ Communication Difficult to Receive

Then, throw the ball rather hard to a student and discuss what happened. Explain that just like a toss in a ball game, a communication message must be sent carefully. You don't want to send the message too loudly because it will be difficult to receive.

Now that you have captured your students' attention and curiosity, they will be prepared to brainstorm and role play to discover what good communicators do. Tell the students that you'll be coming to their room for the next 10 weeks to help them become expert communicators.

Developing the Concept of Brainstorming

Ask students, "What do expert communicators do? Let's brainstorm!" (Prior to actually brainstorming, develop the concept of brainstorming by equating it to a rainstorm, with a downpouring of ideas.) Explain that they'll be observing and participating in a lot of role plays to make these discoveries.

Developing the Concept of Role Playing

Check to see if students are familiar with role playing. Once students understand that brainstorming and role playing will be the structure of the Lab, you and the classroom teacher will begin the role playing so students can discover what good communicators do.

Identifying What Good Communicators Do

Creating Role Plays

Call the students' attention to the poster board with the brainstorm message, "What Do Good Communicators Do?" Explain that you'll be role playing so the students can pinpoint what good communicators do.

With the classroom teacher, begin at the top of the communication vocabulary list and role play *poor communication,* making the communication skill obvious to your students. Welcome students into role plays as soon as possible to get them more actively involved in the learning process. For example, have a conversation with no eye contact. These role plays need to be quick, taking no longer than 30 seconds.

Suggested Role Plays

◆ Eye Contact: Both teachers converse without eye contact.

◆ Observation: You play a parent on the phone, while the classroom teacher plays a child who comes charging up and starts talking to her parent.

◆ Body Language: The classroom teacher plays the role of a parent and you play the child. The parent asks the child to take out the garbage can, and the child takes it out using uncooperative body language.

◆ Listening: You and the classroom teacher talk, and one of you doesn't pay attention to a word the other is saying.

◆ Turn Taking: You and the classroom teacher talk, having one of you keep interrupting the other one.

◆ The *Way*: You and the classroom teacher play two students who are working on math. One student struggles, and the other says, "Oh, that's easy!"

◆ Stay on the Subject: The classroom teacher starts telling a story to the class and keeps changing the subject.

◆ Normal Volume: You start talking too loudly to the class, then too softly.

◆ Normal Pitch: The classroom teacher talks to the class in too high a pitch, then in too low a pitch.

◆ Clear Speech: You mumble to the class so that you are not understood.

◆ Rate of Speech: The classroom teacher starts speed-talking to the class.

◆ Adequate Distance: While standing too close to each other, you and the classroom teacher talk.

◆ Don't Fidget: You fidget to the point of distraction while communicating to the classroom teacher.

This isn't meant to be an exhaustive list of communication skills, but rather some core skills that good communicators use. Feel free to create additional role plays for all of the skills that you and the classroom teacher deem important.

Role plays can easily be created from answering the question, "What's getting in the way of learning and/or positive relationships in the classroom?"

Assessing Role Plays

After each role play, call "freeze" and ask the students what happened. The students will isolate the communication skill you and the classroom teacher didn't use. Next, write the skill that was identified on the poster board and explain how good communicators use eye contact, listening, etc.

When you've listed at least twelve communication skills on the poster board, read them aloud with your students. Then comment that this is a lot to think about when we communicate. Ask the students to identify which communication skills their class is really good at and which ones they want to work on. Recall from the pre-Lab meeting the students' communication strengths and weaknesses as reported by the classroom teacher.

Weekly Communication Classes

Remind your students that you'll be teaching them communication for the next nine weeks (this typically gets a cheer since they've had a ball watching the role plays). Tap into their enthusiasm by asking the following:

> *Why would we want to teach communication in school?*
>
> *How is communication important at school?*
>
> *At home?*
>
> *With friends?*

Your students will naturally have some of their own insights regarding the importance of communication, and they'll gain even more insights from participating in upcoming role plays with their teachers. Let your students know that they're ready to participate in role playing.

School, Friendship, & Home Role Plays

School

Suggest that your students discover how communication can help them in school. Through role playing, your students will become aware of the fact that they can learn faster and enjoy school more when they practice good communication skills. Create role plays that pinpoint problems this particular class is having. For example, students don't listen, they have poor attitudes, and/or they break classroom rules.

Creating Role Plays

For each role play, select a student to play the role of the teacher and others to play students in the class. It's often helpful to select students for the role plays who need to focus on the specific communication skill being taught. For example, a student with poor turn-taking skills would benefit from experiencing being interrupted in a role play. Meanwhile, you and the classroom teacher will take turns playing the parts of students who are poor communicators. The teacher who isn't in the role play will act as the facilitator to debrief the students to determine what happened because of poor communication.

Suggested Role Plays

◆ Don't pay attention during the lesson.

◆ Interrupt the teacher to ask a question that has just been answered.

◆ Have a poor attitude when an assignment is given.

◆ Daydream and distract others while the teacher is teaching.

Assessing Role Plays

Following each role play, call "freeze" and ask your students the following:

Who wasn't a good communicator?

What happened because of poor communication?

How did poor communication make the other students and the teacher feel?

Remember not to debrief for too long as students may lose interest.

Problem Solving

Choose a student to take the role playing teacher's place and invite the group to role play the situation again by using good communication skills. Following the action, call "freeze" and ask your students to explain how using good communication helps in school.

Friendship

In this series of role plays, your students will discover how good communication can make people want to be their friends and to cooperate with them.

Creating Role Plays

Create role plays that pinpoint some of the communication conflicts your students have experienced, such as excluding, teasing, ignoring, and fighting with peers. You and the classroom teacher will join a few students in each role play to play poor communicators so students can realize how important communication is to their friendships.

Suggested Role Plays

- ◆ Someone asks to join your game, and you exclude her.

- ◆ Tease a peer for making a mistake.

- ◆ Tell someone in the group her idea was dumb.

- ◆ Brag about how much better you are than the others.

Assessing Role Plays

Following the action, call "freeze" and ask your students the following:

Who wasn't a good communicator?

What happened because of poor communication?

How did poor communication make people feel?

Problem Solving

Choose a student to take the role playing teacher's place and invite the group to role play the situation again using good communication. Following the action, call "freeze" and ask your students how good communication helps in our friendships.

Home

In this series of role plays, your students will learn how important communication is at home. Recall comments from your students' parents regarding communication conflicts they have at home, such as not giving a younger sister a turn to talk, not pitching in to help, not listening, or not following the rules.

Creating Role Plays

Create role plays where students will play the roles of the parents, and you and the classroom teacher will play the roles of siblings.

Suggested Role Plays

◆ At the dinner table, everyone interrupts.

◆ A parent talks to a child who is glued to the TV set and doesn't respond.

◆ A child complains about doing chores.

Assessing Role Plays

Following each role play, call "freeze" and explore the following with your students:

Who wasn't a good communicator?

What happened because of poor communication?

How did poor communication make people feel?

Problem Solving

Choose a student to take the role-playing teacher's place and invite the group to role play this situation again using good communication. Following the action, call "freeze" and ask your students how good communication helps at home.

```
Notes ✐

```

Wrap Up

"Today we made lots of discoveries about what good communicators do. (Refer to the poster board and read the list out loud with your students.) Each week we'll be working on one of these skills so we can become expert communicators."

Recap the Springboard section of this Lab and remind your students of their communication strengths and the areas that their class decided they wanted to work on in the coming weeks.

How will our improved communication help us at school?

With friends?

At home?

Communication Challenge

Leave your students with a communication challenge. Encourage them to be aware of communication skills they're especially good at. Have them identify communication skills they'd like to improve. Remind students that you'll be teaching a variety of communication skills throughout the program.

Classroom Carryover Activities

1. Communication Reinforcement

Since your students are concentrating on observing their communication, make specific comments about good communication when you observe it by using the vocabulary of CommunicationLab. For example, you might comment, "Good observation, David. You didn't interrupt when I was talking to the principal."

2. Communication Self-Awareness

Remind your students that they should observe their own communication habits. Choose a specific part of the day and ask them to observe how they communicate. At the end of the activity, have your students share their observations about their own and others' good communication.

3. Communication Observation

Invite your students to observe others' communication throughout the day. They can observe their friends at school and in their neighborhood, their parents, siblings, strangers, and even actors on television. After completing their observations, have your students discuss their observations about what good communicators do.

4. Communication Experimentation

Challenge your students to see what happens when they fail to be good communicators. For example, they could communicate without eye contact or they could constantly interrupt. Encourage them to notice the other communicator's reactions. What happened because of poor communication?

Parent Lab

1. **Talk Time**

Create a talk time between your student and his parent(s). Invite family members to think about what makes each of them a good communicator. You might have the family look over the list of communication skills that were generated in the first Lab lesson.

Ask family members to give one another specific praise regarding their communication. For example, a parent might say, "Danny, I appreciate your eye contact when I'm talking. It makes me feel like you're listening."

Have family members ask one another what one skill they would like to see each other improve. Discuss how and where family members will work on developing these communication skills. Have family members practice giving positive feedback as they improve their communication.

2. **Modeling Good Communication**

Remind parents about the value of modeling good communication behavior for their children. Suggest to parents to "play up" or call attention to their own communication behaviors. For example, when a parent wants to talk to his child when he's watching TV, the parent can say, "Matthew, you were watching TV earlier when I wanted to talk to you. I didn't interrupt because my message wasn't urgent."

Have a discussion about the benefits of having parents self-correct their communication behavior in front of their children. For example, a parent might apologize after interrupting her child and then say, "Excuse me, I interrupted you. I'm trying to be a better communicator."

Dear Parents,

Hello! This week, the students in your child's class are improving their awareness and appreciation of good communication. Through role-playing activities, your child discovered what skills good communicators use.

They learned that good communicators:

- use eye contact
- observe before they communicate
- notice body language
- listen
- take turns
- use a polite tone of voice

- speak clearly
- use an appropriate rate of speech
- act interested
- remain on the topic
- allow adequate space between communicators

This list could easily be expanded, but even these 11 skills are a lot to remember when communicating!

To help your child focus on good communication, your family might spend this week noticing all the habits good communicators use. For example, if your daughter accidentally interrupts you and apologizes, you might comment on her good communication.

You may also enjoy having each family member verbally identify his best communication skill. For instance, Dad might be a good turn taker or your son might be a good listener.

Once all family members are aware of communication, enhancing and learning new communication will be much easier.

Sincerely,

Lesson 2:
Observation Skills

The classroom teacher's reading group has just reached a climactic point in the story with students on the edge of their seats, when the teacher feels a tug at her elbow, followed by the predictable refrain, "Ms. Tyler, I don't know how to do this math problem." Ugh. Friday seems light years away. These constant interruptions from students can drive a teacher wild. On certain days, these interruptions may even make a teacher consider going into another profession. Unfortunately, the daily, patient reminder, "Can't you see I'm busy?" doesn't seem to help or to have any carryover from day-to-day.

Classroom teachers aren't alone. Teachers all across the country experience similar daily aggravations and lose valuable teaching time as a result. Why? The truth is that many students have not developed fundamental observation skills. They communicate with poor timing, inappropriately interpret social situations, or are inattentive to the significant nonverbal information that teachers provide throughout the day.

With CommunicationLab, you can help students improve their powers of observation. Classroom teachers will observe students' communication skills grow as a child notes, "Danny is angry, so I won't bother him," or "My teacher is busy, so I'll wait or find out when would be a good time to talk." You'll observe the classroom teacher's relief as he gains increased teaching time, thanks to more observant and considerate student communicators. Over time, you'll also observe the classroom teacher's increased patience with students as students become more considerate communicators.

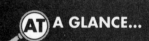 **A GLANCE...**

In this lesson on observation skills, you'll teach your students how to:

◆ use observation skills to help them gain useful academic and social information

◆ read the nonverbal situation before communicating in order to improve the timing and effectiveness of their communication

Vocabulary

observation: looking at a situation before communicating so one can communicate appropriately with good timing

self-improvement: correcting and improving one's performance

say what you see: commenting and questioning about what is observed

Materials

five different kinds of hats

props necessary for the role plays you create

Springboard

Help your students recap the communication skills they learned in the last Lab.

Who can tell me what we learned last time?

What communication skills are you already good at?

Which skills would you like to work on?

"We all know what our strengths are, and each of us has something in mind that we'd like to improve. We call that *working on self-improvement*. We should continually try to be the best people we can by looking critically at ourselves, identifying the things we want to improve, and then working on them. Adults, as well as children, can benefit from working on self-improvement. (Indicate an area of communication that you're good at and an area that needs improvement.)

Warm Up

Note: For students above sixth grade, move directly to the role plays.

Observation

"Today, we're going to learn how our eyes can help us become better communicators. We use our eyes to make observations. In fact, I observe that ...." (Begin by making observations about your students to help them discover both the meaning of the word *observation* and the importance of observing people and situations.) You might say, "I observe that Beth is wearing a green shirt, I observe that Ray is sitting with his hands folded," or "I observe that Genny has a new haircut."

Invite your students to make their own observations by asking a specific student, "What do you observe?" Continue inviting students to make observations by adding the following praise, "Nice observation!"

This Warm Up Activity will solidify the word *observation*, which will serve as a useful tool for the remainder of the school year.

Observation Defined

Next inquire, "Who can tell me what *observation* means?" Your students may use words like *watch, notice,* and *see* to describe observation. Acknowledge their accuracy, "Yes. We notice, see, and watch so we can observe and become better communicators. Are you ready to play an observation game?"

Observation Games

Select one of the following observation activities. Playing observation games will help your students sharpen their observation skills.

1. See If You Can See
   (For younger students)

   Ask your students to identify objects in the classroom with observable features. You might ask them to find something red, round, wooden, metal, shiny, or sharp. Then, challenge your students to find objects that are red and shiny, but not plastic, or something that's blue, but not big.

2. Hats Off #1

Select three to five students to stand in front of the classroom wearing silly hats. (You might choose fewer students when working with younger students.)

Instruct students to closely observe who is wearing which hat because they'll be changing their hats. After your students have made their observations, escort the "Mad Hatters" outside the classroom to swap hats. Back into the class they go so their pals can make their observations!

3. Hats Off #2

You can also play this game by having students line up in two rows facing each other. Label the rows A and B. Students in Row A will wear the hats first, while students in Row B use their observation skills to note who is wearing which hat.

Then, students in Row B will close their eyes so students in Row A can swap hats with each other. Following this hat exchange, Row B's students will make their observations and report where the hats were before and where they are now. Following their success, Row A's students become the observers while students in Row B get to enjoy the fun of wearing and swapping silly hats.

Now your students are ready to enjoy and learn about the importance of observation skills through role playing. Spark their enthusiasm by inquiring, "Are you ready for role playing?" Don't be surprised to hear a unanimous cheer to let the role plays begin!

School, Friendship, & Home Role Plays

School

In the first series of role plays, your students will discover how improved observation skills can help them in school.

First, they'll learn that they must observe before they communicate to ensure appropriate timing. If it's a bad time for them to communicate, they'll make appointments with teachers and parents. This improved communication will be especially useful for the students on your caseload as they interact with better listeners and have less competition, thereby facilitating increased fluency and linguistic functioning.

Creating Role Plays

Recall situations where a student interrupted the teacher because the student didn't observe before he communicated. Choose a student to play the role of the teacher and some other students to play the parts of students in the class. You or the classroom teacher will play the part of a student and will purposely interrupt the teacher.

Suggested Role Plays

◆ The teacher is helping a student, and another student interrupts by asking for help.

◆ The teacher is in deep concentration at her desk correcting papers when a student interrupts from his seat.

◆ Two teachers are having a private conversation when a student barges in to say something.

Assessing Role Plays

Following each blatant interruption, the facilitating teacher will call "freeze" and explore the following:

Who wasn't a good communicator?

What communication skill did the student forget to use?

What happened because the student forgot to observe before he communicated?

How did the student's poor communication make the teacher feel?

What could the interrupter have done instead of interrupting?

Problem Solving

Suggest to your students that if someone is too busy to communicate with them, they can make an appointment for a better time to communicate. You and the classroom teacher can demonstrate this by role playing the same scenario, but this time instead of interrupting, the interrupter will say, "I observe that you are busy. When would be a good time to communicate?"

Making Appointments

Create a few more role plays so your students can practice noticing that the teacher is busy and then making an appointment. This technique of using better timing can have incredible payoffs. Parents and teachers report that even children as young as kindergarten are making appointments to communicate. Adults must remember to let the child know when they're no longer busy to reinforce the child's new communication skill!

Creating Communication Signals

Realistically, students will continue to accidentally interrupt. Following your students' success with making appointments, discuss the idea of creating signals that will remind them to communicate with good timing by asking the following:

What is a signal?

What is the signal used for?

What signal could the classroom teacher give you to remind you to wait before communicating?

(For example, place a finger up to signal them to wait. This signal is generally used when a student accidentally interrupts you. Don't give the student eye contact when you give the signal as this reinforces their interruption.)

What signal could the classroom teacher give you to tell you to go back to your chair until she can get back to you?

(For example, place your entire hand up like a stop sign. Again, don't give the student eye contact. This signal is generally used when a student wants your attention, and you are in the middle of a private conversation.)

Create additional scenarios where students will accidentally interrupt, and the teacher gives the agreed upon signal. Practice using these signals to create a more cooperative, efficient atmosphere. Signals save a tremendous amount of teaching time. This week's Classroom Carryover Activities will give your students additional practice with this new communication technique.

Friendship

In this series of role plays, your students will discover that they can actually make a situation better just because they're present. In addition, they'll learn that commenting and questioning about what they observe (we'll call this *say what you see*) is an excellent way to start a conversation and build rapport.

Creating Role Plays

To initiate this group of role plays, recall situations when a student could have used help or encouragement. Next, invite a student to play this role while one of the teachers *says what she sees.*

Suggested Role Plays

◆ A student is too shy to ask a group to join its game, so one of the players invites the shy student to join the group.

◆ A student gets hurt, someone observes this, and comes to the rescue.

◆ A student is having a noticeably difficult time with his math when someone notices and asks if she can help.

Assessing Role Plays

Call "freeze" following each role play, and discuss how using observation skills made a difference by asking the following questions:

What was said and done to make the situation better?

How did that make everyone feel?

Suggest that commenting and questioning are great ways to start a conversation. For instance, if Uncle Anthony were fixing a bike, what question or comment could you use to start a conversation? Challenge your students with other scenarios to give them practice starting conversations, like the following:

◆ A friend has a new haircut.

◆ A little sister is frustrated because she can't get her shoe tied.

◆ A teacher is walking down the hall with her arms loaded with books.

The classroom teacher can help students further develop this skill during the coming week by using the Classroom Carryover Activities. These carryover suggestions are also an excellent way to enhance your direct therapy sessions with the students on your caseload who may require additional instruction.

Home

In this group of role plays, your students will learn the importance of making observations at home. Recall parents' comments regarding things about which they wish their children would be more aware and considerate, like noticing when parents are busy, tired, upset, or need help.

Creating Role Plays

Now create role plays and ask volunteers to play the roles of the parents. Take turns with the classroom teacher being children who forget to observe while communicating.

Suggested Role Plays

◆ Mom is reading the newspaper when her child comes bounding into the room wanting to discuss his whole day at school.

◆ Dad is busy cooking when his child comes in and rattles off a list of things needed for school the next day.

◆ While Mom is on the phone, her child starts a conversation with her.

◆ The parents, exhausted from a day at work, have their feet up when their children come into the room and start arguing.

◆ Dad is carrying a huge load of laundry and could use some help, but his children walk right past him.

Assessing Role Plays

Following the action, call "freeze" and explore what happened because of poor communication. Ask the following questions:

What happened because observation skills were not used?

How did that make the parents feel?

How could the children have communicated differently?

Problem Solving

Instruct the students to role play the situation again, only this time using their observation skills to ensure good timing. Following the action, call "freeze" and ask your students how observing helped the situation.

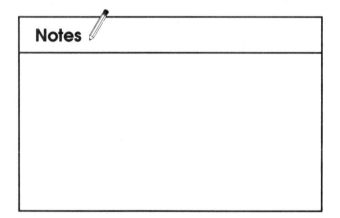

Wrap Up

"What good observers you've been today! Today in CommunicationLab, we learned that observation skills can help us at school, at home, and with our friendships."

Ask the following:

Who can tell me how observation skills help us at school?

At home?

With friends?

"Remember, we can observe when someone is busy and make an appointment so we can communicate with better timing."

Brainstorm by asking the following:

What are some things that I might be doing when you need help from me?

What could you say to make an appointment?

What are some things your parents could be busy with when you want to talk to them?

What could you say to make an appointment?

Communication Challenge

During the next week, have your students observe when someone is busy and then make an appointment to communicate later. Remind students that they'll be asked to share how using their observation skills helped them communicate with better timing and how that made them and the other person feel.

Classroom Carryover Activities

1. Communication Observation

To avoid interrupting, your class has been learning how important it is to observe both the people and the situation while communicating.

One day this week, challenge your students to purposely interrupt an adult and a child. Instruct them to observe what happens to the person who was interrupted, as well as what happens to themselves. At the end of the day, lead a group discussion to crystallize what happens because of interruptions. Some suggested facilitative questions follow:

What did the person that was interrupted do?

How might he have felt?

Do you think he would be a good listener under these circumstances?

Have students tune into what happened to them when they interrupted.

What happened to their speech and how did they feel?

End this activity with a wrap up that reminds your students how important it is to use good timing while communicating.

2. Communication Reinforcement

To reinforce your students' commitment to avoiding interruptions, you must catch your students while they're intentionally waiting to communicate, rather than interrupting. At the beginning of a school day, inform your students that you'll be watching for good observers that day. When you catch someone waiting, rather than interrupting, give her five minutes of "free choice time" at the end of the day, or choose a reinforcement that is more appropriate for your style and classroom. Remember, it's not necessary to give any tangible reinforcement since the verbal praise is extremely motivating.

3. Making Appointments

Your students will benefit from having an additional 10-15 minute practice session making appointments when someone is busy. First, have your students brainstorm a list of occasions when a person was busy and the student wanted to communicate with him. Specifically ask, "What was the busy person doing?" Next, have your students role play these situations to practice making appointments and communicate with better timing.

4. Starting Conversations

Starting conversations is often difficult for people. It can be especially difficult for students with speech and/or language handicaps, so you may wish to provide your students with additional practice starting a conversation by saying what they see.

Invite one student to role play an action, such as doing homework, playing an instrument, or repairing a bike tire. Then, ask another student to start a conversation by saying what they see. For example, "Oh, I didn't know you played the piano!" Your students will both enjoy and benefit from creating numerous role plays for this activity.

Parent Lab

1. **Communicating with Improved Timing**

Work with the family to create a list of reasons the members need to communicate with one another. Next, generate a list of how a family member might be busy when the need to communicate arises.

Through role playing, demonstrate how to observe while approaching a situation so you don't interrupt. Show how to stand an appropriate distance while waiting to communicate. Begin talking when you receive eye contact using a script like, "Mom, are you busy? I want to ask you something."

Debrief to identify the cues that let you know the parent was busy. Give family members practice with this process. Remind everyone to communicate appreciation for not interrupting.

2. **The Signal (Self-Correction)**

Think out loud with parents and their child to list predictable times when a parent is busy and their child needs their attention.

Through role playing, demonstrate how to give the child "the signal" to self-correct after interrupting. Then, reverse roles so parents can practice giving their child the signal following an interruption. Reinforce parents when they signal a child without giving eye contact to the interrupter. Remind parents to give their children immediate feedback for honoring the signal.

Dear Parents,

This week in CommunicationLab, we're focusing on observation skills. Many children fail to make important observations before communicating, and therefore, they interrupt or catch people at a bad time.

Soon you should be observing the same child who used to catch you at a bad time now making an observation like, "Oh, Mom/Dad, I see that you're reading the newspaper. When would be a good time to communicate?" No doubt, you'll be so pleased with your child's good communication that you may be tempted to put down the paper right then and there! While that would reinforce good communication, it would be just as helpful to let your child know when it would be a better time to talk to you. Be sure to follow through with the scheduled meeting!

It would also be helpful to model good observation skills by noticing when your child is busy and then making an appointment to communicate with him/her later. For example, you might say, "I see that you're in the middle of watching a show. When it's over, I'd like to talk to you."

Since you know that your child won't always remember not to interrupt, work together to create a signal that lets your child know you're busy. At school, we're using the universal "wait one minute" signal which we give to students who interrupt. Remember not to give your child eye contact when using the signal as it will reinforce the interruption.

Sincerely,

Lesson 3: Body Language

We're all aware that there are the *words,* and then there is the *message*! We use our entire bodies when communicating. Our faces and bodies are constantly sending messages along with our words. Therefore, it's essential that we not only monitor our own body language, but we also monitor the body language of others.

In fact, FREEZE! What is your body language communicating right now? Yes, you're reading this book, but is your face all tensed up? Someone walking by might think that you're concentrating. Another person might assume that you disagree with what you're reading. And still another may chalk it up to your being in a grumpy mood. The same body language produces three different interpretations, leading to true miscommunication. It happens all the time, not because of the words we use, but because of the message we send with our body language.

Your students are frequently the victims of miscommunication because they often misinterpret another's body language as well as fail to monitor their own body language. For instance, some students assume a teacher doesn't like them because they misread the teacher's body language when the teacher is correcting a mistake on a math assignment. Think of the stuttering child who experiences a block and observes the listener grimacing. You probably have students that are rarely included in a group game because their body language just doesn't look inviting. It's not this child's speech and language that causes her to be excluded from the game, but her negative body language.

Before we open our mouths, people make a first impression by the nonverbal messages we send. When a child has a speech and/or language impairment, it can be even more difficult for him to be accepted by a group, since children are known for teasing. It becomes even more important for children with speech and/or language impairments to learn to send positive body language so their

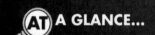
AT A GLANCE...

In this lesson on body language, you'll teach your students how to achieve the following:

◆ to recognize when another student needs thinking time

◆ to monitor their own body language to encourage other learners

◆ to say what they see to confirm or clarify body language and avoid miscommunication

◆ to read the listener's body language to determine if the message is understood

peers will be more likely to include them. Then, any speech and/or language impairment they may have will be less of a handicap because they've been accepted by the group.

In this communication lesson, you'll open a whole new world of communication by moving your students behind the words to observe the nonverbal message or body language. Think about it: what is *not* said often speaks the loudest and is remembered the longest.

Vocabulary

body language: communicating nonverbal messages with facial expressions and body

facial expression: communicating nonverbal messages with one's face

miscommunication: misunderstanding the intended message

thinking time: allowing extra time to process and formulate information

encourage: being supportive and giving confidence

discourage: disapproving or teasing

self-correct: correcting one's errors

monitor: observing and being aware of one's own actions

taking care of yourself: asking for what one needs to assist learning and to protect one's own feelings

check it out: asking for clarification of another's actions or words

Materials

chalkboard

index cards with nonverbal messages printed on them (See the Warm Up Activity.)

props necessary for role plays you create

Springboard

Follow up on last week's Communication Challenge by asking students the following:

Who can tell me what last week's challenge was?

Did you observe someone who was busy and then make an appointment?

How did they react?

Was this helpful to communication?

Would you ever use this communication strategy again?

How else might you use this strategy?

Did you know that you can communicate without even saying a word?

Nonverbal Messages/Body Language

Begin by sending several nonverbal messages (such as "hi, come, stop," or "no") to see if your students can observe and read your nonverbal messages. After each success, you can reinforce the vocabulary of CommunicationLab by saying something like, "You're exactly right. You observed my body language. Can anyone tell me what body language is?"

Invite your students to send a few simple nonverbal messages right from their seats, like "Good job, bad job, okay," or "Don't do that."

Following the group's success, lead them into the Warm Up Activity with reinforcement such as, "You've been sending messages with your body and reading my body language. Sometimes we send messages that aren't so easy to read. Are you ready to play the Body Language Game so you can become even better communicators?"

Warm Up

Body Language Game

On separate index cards, print nonverbal messages for selected students to pantomime while the other students observe and try to interpret. Some nonverbal messages include:

- bored
- in a hurry
- worried
- afraid
- excited
- surprised
- shocked
- lazy
- impatient
- frustrated
- cold
- hot
- hungry
- happy
- daydreaming

Say What You See

You'll want some of these nonverbal messages to be difficult to interpret immediately so your students can learn how to observe and then say what they see by checking it out. For example, one nonverbal pantomime could be to use body language that suggests that someone is concentrating. This activity not only teaches your students the concept of miscommunication, but it will provide them with the tools to avoid miscommunication.

Invite one student to the front of the classroom to send a nonverbal message while a selected student reads the body language from her seat.

Check It Out

When the observers say what they see, ask them if they're sure. For example, encourage them to say what they see and then check it out by saying something like, "You look bored. Are you bored?" The person sending the non-

verbal message can either confirm or clarify by saying, "No, I'm not bored. I'm just thinking."

Miscommunication and Monitoring

This is a perfect opportunity to teach the concept of miscommunication. Explain that sometimes we're unaware of what message our body language is sending, so we need to monitor our body language. Ask the class, "Can anyone tell me what *monitor* means?"

Continue the game until the students understand the importance of talking about what they see so they can read the full message behind the words and, thereby, avoid miscommunication.

Now that your students are focused on seeking the full understanding of a message by reading and monitoring body language, they're ready to participate in the role plays. You and the classroom teacher may choose to create your own role plays to fit your students' particular needs.

As your students become familiar and comfortable with role playing, they may have some suggestions of their own. When students start suggesting their own ideas for role plays, be reassured that CommunicationLab has taken hold, and your students are becoming active learners and problem solvers. Congratulations!

School, Friendship, & Home Role Plays

School

Role Play 1
Thinking Time

Explain that many people need extra time to think about what they want to say before they say it. It's helpful when people around them use body language that communicates patience, support, understanding, and acceptance. Find out when your students need extra thinking time. Is it when called on in class, when writing answers, when solving math problems, or when talking with unfamiliar people? Your students' experiences will serve as a good springboard to create role plays, or you may choose to use one of the following suggested role plays. In this series of role plays, you'll teach your students how to give others thinking time and how to ask for it themselves.

Creating Role Plays

For each role play, select a student to role play a situation in which she needs extra thinking time. You might wish to choose a student who actually requires that extra bit of time for processing and formulating language. Meanwhile, you or the classroom teacher can play the part of an impatient communicator.

Suggested Role Plays

◆ A teacher calls on a student in class to answer a question.

◆ A student tries to remember an important message his parents wanted him to give the teacher.

◆ A student verbally tries to solve a math word problem with a peer.

Assessing Role Plays

Following each role play, call "freeze," and debrief with your students by asking the following:

Who wasn't a good communicator?

What did this person's body language communicate?

Now explore with the student who was involved in the role play how the teacher's body language made the student feel. Ask her

if this kind of body language encouraged or discouraged her.

Problem Solving

Invite another student to role play the same scenario, but this time tell her to send body language that will encourage the other student to take the thinking time she needs. After their success with this role play, suggest to the thinking student that she talk about, and ask for what she needs by saying something like, "I need some extra thinking time."

This scenario will no doubt be familiar and helpful to many of the students on your caseload since they often have a difficult time finding words or speaking fluently. This is a natural opportunity to ask the class if anyone has ever experienced someone sending them impatient body language. Ask the following:

How did the impatient body language affect them?

What did the students do?

After students verbalize their discouraging experiences, encourage them to choose a friend to help them role play the situation so they can problem solve. Ask how they can give and ask for thinking time when it's needed.

Explain that asking for thinking time is a way of taking care of yourself because you're asking for what you need. Many of your students will need additional encouragement to take care of themselves and will need teachers and peers to remind them to ask for thinking time. This help is best offered through observations and comments from the teacher such as, "Looks like you need some thinking time," or "Do you want some thinking time?" This subtle reminder will give your students the anchor they need to remind them that it's okay to take time to respond.

Role Play 2
Observing Body Language

Teach your students how to observe the listener's body language to make sure that their message is being understood.

Creating Role Plays

Have the classroom teacher role play several different short conversations with various students, sending different facial expressions in each conversation to communicate the following.

Suggested Role Plays

◆ You didn't understand the speaker.

◆ You agree with what is being said.

◆ You disagree with what is being said.

◆ You're bored with the conversation.

Assessing Role Plays

Call "freeze" after each role play. Ask the speaker about the facial expressions he observed.

What does the listener's body language mean?

Knowing what this body language means, what should you do?

Problem Solving

If necessary, role play this scenario again and observe how your students "repair" or adjust the communication after observing the listener's body language. Some of your students may need you to facilitate this activity. Point out the listener's body language and help the speaker respond appropriately. You and the classroom teacher can model additional suggestions to expand your students' repertoire for repairing conversations. For example, when

you observe that the listener looks puzzled, you might ask, "Am I being unclear?"

Friendship

Role Play 1
Monitoring Body Language

Your students are constantly sending and receiving messages that encourage or discourage self esteem, and that affect them academically and socially. In this part of the Lab, your students will learn how to monitor body language as well as how to problem solve when they receive discouraging body language from others.

Creating Role Plays

Create role plays that pinpoint some of the discouraging nonverbal messages students send each other. Often these messages will cause peers to shut down academically and may prevent them from verbally risking in the classroom.

In these role plays, your students will act out making common mistakes, while you and the classroom teacher take turns playing the part of another student who sends discouraging body language.

Suggested Role Plays

◆ A student mispronounces a word, and someone makes fun of him.

◆ A student gives a wrong answer and is mocked.

◆ A student is on the wrong page when the teacher calls on her, and the class laughs.

Assessing Role Plays

Following the action, call "freeze" and explore these questions with your students:

What did your body language communicate?

How will this affect the learner?

Has anyone ever made a mistake and experienced someone making fun of them with their body language?

Problem Solving

Invite your students to create role plays with their friends to show what it looked like when someone made fun of them. Challenge your students to problem solve to arrive at different ways they can respond if this should happen again in real life.

Our body language communicates, so we need to use it to encourage, not discourage, our friends. Teach your students that this is called *monitoring*. When we catch ourselves sending discouraging body language, we can self-correct.

Ask if any of your students know what *self-correct* means. Model self-correction by sending negative body language and then changing it. For example, if you interrupted someone, you could apologize and then let him have his turn. When you and the classroom teacher observe students self-correcting, comment, "Good self-correction. You wanted to encourage, not discourage, your friend." If a student needs to be reminded to self-correct, he now understands the vocabulary so you can prompt by saying, "You need to self-correct your body language to be more encouraging."

Role Play 2
Facing Discouraging Body Language

Provide an opportunity for your students to problem solve when the members of a group

they want to join send discouraging body language.

Creating Role Plays

Launch this group of role plays by asking your students if they have ever wanted to join a group game, but they knew the group didn't want to include them. Create role plays from your students' ideas, situations you have observed, or from the following suggestions. You and the classroom teacher can take turns being the communicator who sends the discouraging message.

Suggested Role Plays

◆ Someone asks to join a game and the group members send discouraging nonverbal messages.

◆ With your body language, tell someone in front of a group that his idea is dumb.

◆ Let someone join the game, only give her "dirty looks," or just plain ignore her.

Assessing Role Plays

Following the action, call "freeze" and ask your students these questions:

Who wasn't a good communicator?

How did the group's body language make them feel?

Problem Solving

Inquire to see if any of your students have ever been sent discouraging body language by a group of their peers. Form a group to role play what this teasing looked like so you can help the students problem solve. You may be surprised to discover that your students have many more helpful suggestions for their peers than we can offer them. In fact, you may find that you and the classroom teacher are talking less as your students begin to take a more active role in the Lab. You'll find this to be especially true of your older students.

Home

Parents often talk about the bad attitudes of kids these days. Negative body language contributes to their understandable frustration with kids' nonverbal communication. The following role plays will help your students become aware of the body language they're sending to their families.

Creating Role Plays

Begin by asking your students if they like to help their parents at home. Which jobs are their least favorite? Now create role plays where a student is the parent and you are the child. The parent asks the child to help, and the child says "Yes" with her words, while simultaneously sending negative body language.

Suggested Role Plays

◆ The parent asks the child to take the garbage out and the child says, "Okay," while ripping it out of his parent's hands and stomping off.

◆ The parent asks the child to help clear the table and the child says, "Okay," but bangs the dishes around while cleaning up.

Assessing Role Plays

Following the role play, call "freeze" and debrief your students by asking the following:

Who wasn't a good communicator?

What did your body language communicate?

What will the parent do because of this body language?

Problem Solving

Extend this role play by asking your students if there is another way to communicate to a parent when you don't want to do something. List your students' suggestions on the chalkboard. Invite your students to role play these options. Teach them that combining words with good body language will help people understand how you're feeling and, therefore, to want to cooperate with you more frequently.

Be prepared for some students to discuss the reality that just because you're positive doesn't mean that others will cooperate with you. Agree with them. It's true. We cannot control anyone else's behavior but our own. The good news is that we're in control of our own behavior and can, therefore, choose to communicate in the most positive, cooperative manner we can. Remind your students that very often we get what we give.

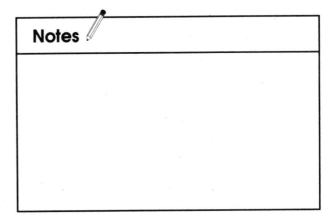

Notes

Wrap Up

"Today in CommunicationLab, we learned that we communicate with more than just our words. We communicate with our . . . (pause so your students can insert the words *body language*). That's right, we communicate with our body language. We also learned that our body language can either encourage or discourage other people."

Ask your students the following:

What are some discouraging messages we send at school with our body language?

What are some encouraging messages?

What are some discouraging messages we send to our families and to our friends?

What are some encouraging messages?

Communication Challenge

Challenge your students to observe and send encouraging body language that communicates caring and a willingness to cooperate and to understand messages. Have students report their findings the next time you meet.

Classroom Carryover Activities

1. Body Language Awareness Day

Help your class become even more tuned into the nonverbal world of communication by creating a *Body Language Awareness Day.*

At the beginning of the school day, gather your students together to discuss body language. Remind them of their discoveries about sending and receiving encouraging and discouraging body language. Encourage your students to observe how other people's body language makes them feel.

At the end of the day, provide an opportunity for your students to share their observations. Help them discover the power of a simple smile.

2. Body Language Clues

Before a lesson, explain to your students that you'll be using extra body language to give clues to the meaning of new vocabulary words. As you use vocabulary that is unfamiliar to your students, use nonverbal clues to help them gain information.

Following your nonverbal clue, say "Freeze! Who can guess from my body language what the word *combine* means? Good, you read my body language to help you learn a new word."

Continue the lesson in this manner to encourage your students to read body language in order to gain academic information.

3. Thinking Time

During a group interactive lesson, remind your students about thinking time. Tell them that during today's reading lesson, they should observe when a friend needs thinking time and then monitor their body language to make sure that they're patiently waiting for their friend to come up with the answer. Encourage your students to ask for thinking time when they need it. When a student requires thinking time during a lesson, comment on students who are sending positive body language.

4. Body Language Encouragement

Before a lesson, remind your students how to monitor their body language if someone makes a mistake. During the lesson, comment when people don't laugh or call negative attention to their peers' errors. Use the vocabulary of CommunicationLab to cue your students. For instance, you might say, "I observed how you all encouraged Zachary when he made a mistake." You may also want Zachary to make his own observations about his friends' body language by asking him if these nonverbal messages were encouraging or discouraging. Then, suggest that Zachary give his friends some positive feedback like, "Thanks for the encouragement!"

Parent Lab

1. Say What You See

Help parents and their children become more aware and accurate when reading each other's body language. Label index cards with various emotions, like frustrated, excited, worried, and bored. Invite one person to choose a card and communicate the emotion through his body language. You can demonstrate how to "say what you see and check it out." For example, you might say, "You look upset. Are you upset?" Invite all family members to send and read body language.

Following the above activity, discuss the importance of body language. Suggest that parents frequently talk about family members' body language. Demonstrate for parents how they can encourage their child to read each other's body language. For example, parents can encourage their child, "Look at my face. What am I communicating?" Remind parents to monitor their tone of voice to be encouraging rather than authoritative.

2. Matching Body Language

For children having difficulty matching their body language to their verbal message, suggest the following technique.

When a child's body language doesn't match his verbal message, demonstrate how parents can ask their child to communicate again (re-role play). For example, when a child looks upset, but his body language conveys that he's happy, a parent can say, "Lamont, I know you're upset, but you don't look upset."

Some children may require a parent to model what *upset* would look like. Other children may benefit from mirror work. Following the parent's demonstration, have the child imitate the body language so his words mirror his body language.

Dear Parents,

Following our communication lesson last week, have you noticed that your child has been using his observation skills more efficiently? Great!

Often it's our body language, our nonverbal messages, that cause poor communication and confrontation. For instance, think about a time when you asked your child to take out the garbage or complete some chore, and she did it, but her body language made you furious!

This week in CommunicationLab, your child learned how to send and receive nonverbal messages or body language. Your child will be using his observation skills to read and monitor body language so he can become more aware of nonverbal messages.

First, your child learned how to monitor her own body language. Then, she learned how to communicate patience when a speaker needs thinking time. At home, if you see your child struggling to find words, take the opportunity to check your body language to make sure that you're communicating that it's all right for her to take thinking time to find the right words. To reinforce this communication skill, ask your child about thinking time. Does she need it? When? How will you know when she needs it?

Next, your child learned how to say what he sees to avoid miscommunication. For example, your child might say, "You look mad." You might respond, "Actually, I was just thinking." Next time you see that your child looks frustrated when doing his homework, you might say what you see, "You look frustrated. Do you need thinking time, or would you like help?"

Your child also learned how to observe a listener's facial expression to determine whether her message was being understood. The next time your child's message is unclear, you can help her by commenting, "Honey, look at my facial expression. I'm unclear about what you and your friends did after school. Can you say it in a different way, please?"

We hope you're observing a lot of encouraging communication at home!

Sincerely,

Lesson 4: Listening

How many times do I have to tell you?

Am I talking to a brick wall?

Hello, anybody home?

Earth calling Mars?

In one ear and out the other!

Sound familiar? We've all either used or heard these listening expressions uttered at the peak of aggravation resulting from having to repeat ourselves because someone wasn't listening. Although these expressions make the point that we're understandably annoyed and want the person to listen, it doesn't provide our students with information on how to listen. That's right, how to listen.

Admittedly, most of us don't need to stop to think about the specific behaviors or habits that good listeners use since listening comes instinctively to most of us. Interestingly, however, there are other people who don't know how to listen and, therefore, need to be taught. It's surprising that few educational curricula specifically teach students these listening behaviors.

We SLP's observe the result of this lack in the curriculum because we see many students on our caseloads who have difficulty maintaining eye contact, asking clarifying questions, or responding to and following directions. In fact, these "poor listening" behaviors are frequently the reason a student is referred to the SLP in the first place.

With this communication lesson, you'll teach the entire class the *how* of listening. Your students will learn how to use these listening habits to improve their comprehension. Your students will also identify what makes it difficult for them to listen, and then they'll problem solve to overcome these listening challenges. Additionally,

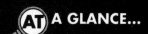
AT A GLANCE...

In this lesson on listening, you'll teach your students the following:

◆ to become aware of the importance of being a good listener

◆ to learn and use the habits of a good listener

◆ to activate listening when faced with competing forces

◆ to secure good listening habits from others

your students will learn ways they can encourage other people to be more active listeners when students are speaking to them.

When your students begin using these improved listening habits, like eye contact, head nods, listening noises, and commenting and questioning on the subject, the classroom teacher will naturally feel more willing to invest extra teaching time, which will provide repetition for students with comprehension problems. After all, who would you rather repeat yourself to, a student who is turned around in her chair daydreaming or a student who is looking at you nodding his head up and down, but needs to hear the message a second time to completely understand what you said?

Vocabulary

listening: seeking understanding by using the habits of a good listener

head nods: acknowledging the speaker by shaking one's head

listening noises: acknowledging that one is following the speaker's train of thought by voicing an occasional, "Oh, Umm," or "M-hmm"

on the subject: contributing to a conversation on the subject

paraphrasing: rewording or repeating back what one understood the speaker to say

talk about talking: talking about talking by saying things like, "I'm listening, but I can't look at you right now because I'm busy"

Materials

favorite short story book

poster board or butcher paper for brainstorming the *Habits of Good Listeners*

props necessary for the role plays you create

Springboard

"Your body language communicates that you're ready for and excited about this week's CommunicationLab!

Did anyone observe or send encouraging body language since our last CommunicationLab?

How did that make you feel?

Did anyone need thinking time or observe someone else who needed it?

Very good, you're all becoming expert communicators with both your words and your body language."

(For older students, proceed to the "Observing Listening Habits" section.)

Listening

"Shhh ... tell me what you hear. Let's name all of the sounds we can hear in and out of our classroom."

Begin calling on students so they can share the sounds they hear, such as the lights buzzing, someone tapping a pencil, people in the hall, or people breathing. Then, call "freeze" and ask, "What do you think we're going to learn about in this week's CommunicationLab? You're exactly right—listening!"

Note: Younger students will love the fact that they guessed what your lesson is. Now they'll be ready to be led into one of the suggested listening warm up games.

Warm Up

Clap When You Hear the Word *Fruitloop*

Choose one of your class's favorite stories that has colorful pictures and loads of action. Tell your students that you're going to read them a story, and every time you say the word *fruitloop,* they should clap their hands. Some classes enjoy hiccuping rather than clapping, which makes this activity even sillier. Begin the story and you'll see your students not only enjoying the fact that they're good listeners, but they'll also get a kick out of how nonsensical the story becomes!

What Will I Ask You To Do?

Another fun listening game is "What will I ask you to do?" In this listening game, you can either tell your students a personal story or choose a book that is a classroom favorite. Warn your students that as you tell the story, you'll be inserting directions they should follow. For instance, you might say, "This morning on the way to work, I saw a ... everybody stand up."

This nonsense listening game will activate your students' listening skills. Following their success with the Warm Up Activity, tell them they're ready to make some discoveries about what good listeners actually do.

Good Listening Habits

"Terrific listening! Now that you're all warmed up, you're ready to make some discoveries about the habits good listeners use. Can anyone tell me what a *habit* is? That's right, a habit is something that we learn to do, like saying 'Please' when asking for a favor. Let's discover the habits that good listeners use."

For Younger Students

Conduct the following two activities as a group with you and the classroom teacher conversing in front of the class, modeling both good and poor listening habits. Help your students identify the habits of good and poor listeners by asking them a facilitative question, such as, "Who can tell me what I did with my eyes while I was listening?" Write their discoveries on the poster board or butcher paper labeled "Habits of Good Listeners."

Observing Listening Habits

Pair your students. Ask each pair to choose one person to be the talker and the other to be the listener. Tell them to get into a two-minute conversation about a chosen topic, such as their first memory of school or their favorite birthday party. Tell the listeners to be the best listeners they know how to be. The talker's job is to observe all the listening habits that the listener uses.

Following this two-minute discovery activity, brainstorm with your students to pinpoint all the habits they observed the listener using. Write these specific observations on the poster board titled "Habits of Good Listeners". (Leave the poster board in the classroom to activate the students' listening habits during the coming weeks.) These listening habits will include:

◆ eye contact

◆ sitting still

◆ not doing more than one thing at a time

◆ smiling

◆ leaning forward

◆ acting interested

◆ nodding one's head

◆ making listening noises like "Oh" and "Umm"

◆ responding, commenting, and questioning on the subject

To wrap up this activity and emphasize the complexity of listening, read aloud all the listening habits that your students have discovered during the Lab. Comment on how much there is to remember when listening.

Poor Listening Skills

Ask your students if they ever forget to listen. Then, invite two students to role play situations to show what poor listening looks like. Have one student model a poor listening habit and the other experience the consequences. Have the students role play behaviors like daydreaming, fidgeting, acting bored, and changing the subject.

For Older Students

Your older students may enjoy giving each poor listening habit a name, such as daydreaming or clock-watching. This labeling will also give your students a vocabulary to use in the future to cue each other when they, in fact, are being a daydreamer or a clock-watcher instead of a good listener. (You and the classroom teacher may wish to target various students who are poor listeners to be talkers so they can experience what happens as a result of poor listening.)

After each role play, help your students discover the consequences that poor listening has on communication. You can begin by asking the talker the following:

What happened to your speech when no one was listening?

How did poor listening make you feel?

Now that your students have a clear picture of what they can actually do to be good listeners, they are ready to participate in role plays

designed to develop their listening habits for school, home, and peer relations.

School, Friendship, & Home Role Plays

School

Role Play 1
Difficulty Listening
Creating Role Plays

Even though your students know what good listeners do, sometimes it's difficult for them to listen because of the daily distractions that occur around them. Since we can predict that distractions will be a part of the learning environment, the first set of role plays will give your students an opportunity to learn how to problem solve when other forces are competing with their listening. The second group of role plays will help provide students with some active listening strategies for the classroom.

For Younger Students

You and the classroom teacher will role play the various distractions that occur in the classroom (see suggestions on the next page). Next, invite a volunteer to participate in a re-role play that demonstrates a solution to the problem. In some cases, you may have to give students a solution and then help them practice using it in the role play.

For Older Students

Begin the role plays by saying something like, "We can see that everyone is familiar with what good listeners do, but does anyone ever have a hard time listening in school? Why?" No doubt you'll get responses like the following:

- Someone is reading aloud while I'm thinking.

- Someone is tapping her pencil.

- Someone is trying to talk to me while I'm supposed to be doing my social studies.

Your students' suggestions will help you create meaningful role plays to teach them how to problem solve under these conditions.

Following each explanation of what makes it difficult to listen, invite the student to create a role play with her peers to show the rest of the class what this distraction looks like. Discuss options for handling distractions or competing forces when your students are trying to listen. Then, have your students role play these options.

Suggested Role Plays

- Someone is bothering a student who is trying to listen.

- Someone is tapping a pencil or making other distracting noises.

- Someone is trying to get a student's attention while the student is trying to listen to the teacher.

Assessing Role Plays

Following the action, call "freeze" and explore the following with your students:

What made it difficult to listen?

Has this ever happened to anyone before?

What did you do to make it easier to listen?

How have other people handled these problems?

Problem Solving

Challenge your students to role play one of the proposed solutions to the suggested problem. Continue to have various groups of students role play other solutions they think may help the situation when someone is distracting them from listening.

After exhausting all solutions, ask your students the following:

Which solution do you think would work for you? Why?

Your students will soon discover how to take care of themselves by moving to another seat, asking a peer to be quiet, or getting a teacher's help when they're struggling to listen. This kind of role-playing activity will leave your students with a repertoire of strategies to overcome distractions so they can be better listeners in school.

Role Play 2
Asking Questions/Paraphrasing

These role plays will teach students how to ask questions and/or paraphrase to increase their comprehension and to activate their listening behaviors.

Creating Role Plays

Invite a student to play the teacher who will teach a lesson while you and the classroom teacher play the role of students to demonstrate what happens when students don't listen while the teacher is teaching. Use either of the following suggested role plays to demonstrate poor listening.

Suggested Role Plays

- Go off the subject while the teacher is teaching.

◆ Be unprepared when the teacher calls on you.

Assessing Role Plays

Now call "freeze!" Use the following questions to debrief your students on their observations about what poor listening did to the lesson:

What did poor listening do to the teacher's lesson?

How do you think this makes the teacher feel?

What does a teacher usually do when students aren't listening?

Do you know how a teacher knows if you're listening?

This is a good opportunity to teach your students that they need to actively participate by letting the teacher know that they're listening and that they either understand or need more information. Do this by teaching your students to either paraphrase what they hear or ask questions if they don't understand. These two active listening habits will help your students either clarify or verify what they hear. Some classes may need you and the classroom teacher to demonstrate paraphrasing and asking questions.

Problem Solving

Invite a few students to use the suggested active listening habits of paraphrasing and questioning while the teacher teaches. Following this second role play, discuss how the results were different because students were listening.

Friendship

People who go through life feeling unheard often grow angry or feel that they have little of importance to say. In the next set of role plays, you'll teach your students how to listen to each other in a way that communicates that they care!

Creating Role Plays

In this set of role plays, you and the classroom teacher will act the parts of students who have poor listening behaviors when playing and talking with other students.

Suggested Role Plays

When a student is telling you something important, do one of the following:

◆ Act bored.

◆ Look at your watch.

◆ Change the subject.

Assessing Role Plays

Following each role play, call "freeze" and explore the following with your students:

How did your poor listening make the other person feel?

What message were you really sending him?

What can you do or say if someone isn't listening?

Problem Solving

Role play the previous situation again, but this time, the student playing the teacher will try to get you to improve your listening behavior. You might suggest to the student to ask if it's a good time to communicate or to have the student let you know how your behavior is making her feel.

Home

We live in such busy times that sometimes it's necessary for us to listen and to do something else at the same time. The problem with this is that often our inability to drop what we're doing to give someone our full attention communicates that we don't care what the person is saying, which can lower his self-esteem. In reality, this is usually not the message the listener intended to send the speaker.

In the next set of role plays, teach your students to talk about talking, saying something like, "I'm listening, but I can't look at you because I need to do something else at the same time. I'm especially busy right now."

Creating Role Plays

Begin by asking your students to recall times when they were busy and someone needed them to listen. After these descriptions, you and the classroom teacher can explain that this also happens to you. Model the concept of talking about talking when you're unable to give your full attention to the student who is talking. For example, you might say, "I'm listening, but I need to keep filing these papers."

Suggested Role Plays

◆ You're busy organizing your desk.

◆ You're busy dusting the furniture.

◆ You're busy filing papers.

Assessing Role Plays

Call "freeze" after each role play and ask your students the following questions:

How did it make you feel when I couldn't give you my full attention?

Did it help to talk about talking?

Problem Solving

Extend this activity by recalling when your students said they couldn't give a teacher, parent, or friend their full attention. Challenge your students to role play these situations to practice talking about talking. Then, encourage your students to teach their parents how to talk about talking when they are unable to drop what they're doing to give someone their full attention. Emphasize that just because a person can't drop what she's doing doesn't mean she doesn't care. Likewise, explain that if there is an emergency, then it's appropriate to give someone your full attention. Brainstorm a list of emergencies that would require an attentive listener.

Notes

Wrap Up

"Today in CommunicationLab, we discovered what good listeners do."

What are some listening habits your class is already good at?

Which listening habits would you like to work on?

(Add your own suggestions to the list.)

"We also learned how good listening can make people feel that we care. We also learned that it's not always easy to listen when we get busy."

When are some times when you feel you're good listeners at school? At home?

81

When can you challenge yourself to use some of our new listening habits?

Begin the Wrap Up by praising your students for actively listening. Ask students how you can let them know how much you appreciate their active listening next time you observe it. Students will often want to create a signal rather than have the teacher stop the lesson and verbally praise. Likewise, the teacher will want to create a signal with her class to remind them to turn on their good listening habits when they seem to forget. For example, you might say, "Class," and point to your ear.

Communication Challenge

Challenge your students to take their new communication skills home to their families. Have them teach their families how to talk about talking when the members are too busy to drop what they're doing and give their full attention to listening.

To help families learn, have your students talk about talking the next time their parents need to talk to them when they're busy. For example, let's say a student is doing her homework, and her stepdad comes in and wants to tell her about his work day. How could she talk about talking? That's right, she could say, "I'm in the middle of my homework. I'm listening, but I can't look at you." She may be surprised to see her parents begin talking about talking.

Classroom Carryover Activities

1. Talk About Talking

When your students are doing independent seat work, and you're grading papers or preparing lesson plans, model talking about talking as students come to your desk to speak with you. For example, you might say, "I'm listening, but I can't look at you because I'm grading papers."

2. Signal for Listening

Before a chosen lesson, remind your students of the signal that praises good listening and the one that reminds them to use their good listening habits. During the lesson, use the signals as appropriate. After the lesson, debrief with students to determine whether these signals were useful to them. Do any changes need to be made?

3. Paraphrasing and Questioning

Before a lesson, remind your students about the role play where they learned how to ask questions and paraphrase to show they were listening and to gain a better understanding of the lesson. Have each student make a personal goal of a certain number of times she'll try to paraphrase and/or question during the upcoming lesson. It's helpful if you tell your students to write their personal goals down so they can see if they accomplished their goals following the lesson.

4. I'm All Ears

For Younger Students

Have students get in a group. Then, ask a volunteer to come to the front of the class to share an experience or to tell about a special toy. Instruct the rest of the group to use as many of the good listening habits as they can while the speaker is talking. When the speaker has finished sharing, ask the speaker what good listening habits he observed in his classmates.

For Older Students

Invite your students to get into pairs and have a two-minute conversation about an academic subject they just learned or a story they recently read. Remind your students to use the good listening habits that are listed on the poster board from the previous CommunicationLab. Then, have them switch partners and pick a personal topic on which to practice their new improved listening skills. Following each two-minute conversation, have the partners tell each other which good listening habits they observed and how it made them feel when their friend listened to them.

Parent Lab

1. Talk Time

Create a talk time for families as an arena to improve listening skills. Encourage a parent and her child to have a five-minute conversation. First, have the child be the speaker and talk about anything. The parent's task is to be a good listener. Remind the child to observe his parent's listening during his "talk time."

After the five-minute conversation, have the child report two positive things that the parent did to show the child she was listening. Also have the child discuss one thing he would like his parent to do to improve her listening. For example, a child might report that he likes when he gets eye contact and when his parent stops what she's doing when the child is talking. The child might also like his parent not to ask too many questions.

Reverse roles so the child can practice listening and the parent can give constructive feedback to help the child become a better listener.

Then, instruct each family member to choose one place during the day to practice listening. Challenge family members to practice working on the one behavior that will help them be better listeners. Remind family members to give each other positive feedback as they modify their listening behaviors.

2. Listening At Home

Listening in the home is challenging because a lot of daily communication happens when family members are in different rooms. Often, a family member ends up talking to people who are busy and aren't even aware they're being spoken to.

Ask family members if they ever need each other's attention when they're in different rooms in their home. Can they effectively communicate this way? This communication exercise will help family members move into the same room when communication calls for active listening.

Next, think out loud with family members to create two lists. On one list, identify where a parent and child might be when they need to communicate with each other. On the other list, identify reasons family members might need to communicate with one another.

Create role plays using the scenarios on the lists to give family members opportunities to observe you role play both the speaker and the listener. (Have the parent help you.) Provide family members with an opportunity to practice being both the listener and speaker.

Role of the speaker

◆ Call family member by name. Don't repeat the name, but call once and wait for a response.

◆ Don't give a direction or begin talking until a family member is in sight.

◆ Smile and praise the family member for coming after hearing his name.

◆ Begin talking.

Role of the listener

◆ Come when your name is called and ask, "Did you call my name?"

◆ Listen to the speaker.

◆ Follow the direction, if one was given.

To wrap up this activity, think out loud with family members to pinpoint a time of day they'll practice this communication exercise. It's important to have a time to practice, as it's unrealistic to expect family members to practice this new behavior all day.

Dear Parents,

How many times have you reached the end of your fuse because you felt your child wasn't listening? Do you hear yourself saying things like, "How many times do I have to tell you? Do I have to repeat myself again?" or "I feel like I'm talking to a brick wall!"

Teachers and parents can relate to the growing frustration that results from all the repeating they have to do when someone doesn't listen the first time.

This week in CommunicationLab, your child learned what it means to be a good listener. Ask your child to recall some of these listening habits and talk about which habits she observes you using. In turn, praise your child for the good listening habits you observe her using. Examples of good listening habits include:

- ◆ eye contact
- ◆ head nods
- ◆ asking questions on the subject
- ◆ commenting and acting interested

You might also want to discuss how each of you could improve your listening skills.

Your child also learned how busy life is and how it's not always possible for people to drop what they're doing to give us their full attention. Your child did learn about the importance of talking about talking (that is, to say that we can't drop what we're doing, but that we're still listening). We challenged the children to teach this new skill at home.

Most importantly, we discussed how when we listen to others, we're communicating that we care.

Our lives are often so busy that it's vital that we look at our own communication to see what messages our listening habits are sending the people we love.

Sincerely,

Lesson 5: Turn Taking

Turn taking! When we think about it, almost everything we do that involves more than one person requires that we wait for our turn. For children, as well as for some adults, waiting is difficult because people are usually eager to be first.

Since we obviously can't be first all the time, what is it that encourages us to wait our turn? Lines certainly help! Lines are probably the "training wheels" of turn taking because they're a visual and structured way to prove whose turn is next.

A comical example of how lines help turn taking comes from an observation I made while watching a group of five ducks swimming in a line. Actually, there were four ducks in line and one lone duck swimming alongside the group. As you can guess, this bold duck was trying to beat the system and budge in between ducks number two and three. Well, duck number two wasn't phased, but duck number three was losing feathers over this unacceptable entry, and he "beaked" the intruder out of the way. Unwilling to give up, the bold duck tried to swim between ducks number three and four to avoid being last. Now guess which duck didn't care? Duck number three of course, because who cares if someone budges in behind you? Now it was duck number four who was defending its cherished position, and the unruly duck was given the mighty beak again!

I share this story because it clearly illustrates this universal issue of turn taking. We all know people who behave like that duck—that is, people who interrupt conversations, who do the majority of the talking, who rarely ask others' for their opinion, who budge into a line, or who don't willingly share.

Our children spend enormous amounts of energy struggling with this concept of waiting for their turn and with the issue of fairness. How often do we find ourselves refereeing whose turn it is, remind-

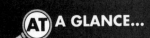

AT A GLANCE...

In the following lesson on turn taking, you'll teach your students how to:

◆ take turns in conversations and in group activities

◆ use effective strategies to enter and exit conversations

◆ surrender when two people start talking at once

◆ hook other people into the conversation

◆ include other people, rather than exclude them

ing students to give someone else a turn, as well as reminding students to include everyone? A lot of valuable teaching time is lost in our daily efforts to manage turn taking.

In this week's CommunicationLab, you'll teach your students exactly what turn taking is and why it's important for learning and for friendships. They'll also learn how to get in and out of conversations without interrupting.

Entering and exiting conversations is a particularly difficult task for a child with weaker verbal skills, especially when he has to compete for a turn. Participation in this CommunicationLab will give these verbally less aggressive students the tools they need to get into social and academic conversations, as well as to help them get involved in games and class projects.

On the other hand, your verbally aggressive students (the "talkers" in the group) will learn how to monitor the number of turns they're taking so everyone gets a chance to participate. Likewise, students will learn how to surrender when two people begin talking at once, as well as how to "hook" the person who surrendered his turn back into the conversation. Your students will also learn how to observe so they can include their peers. You'll also give your students the tools they need to become aware of when they forget to take turns, and how to self-correct so they can continue to participate with good turn taking, which will encourage other people to value their input.

What a difference it will make when your students are taking turns and actually seeking everyone's participation. The class will function more smoothly with a cooperative, caring attitude echoing throughout the classroom. This improved communicative climate will encourage your students to verbally risk and to participate to their fullest. As you observe these significant communication changes, you'll begin to wish that your family and friends could participate in a CommunicationLab

since some of the simplest concepts, like turn taking, can make enormous differences in all of our daily interactions.

Vocabulary

include: encouraging others to participate

exclude: purposely omitting others from participating

budge: cutting in front of someone

interrupt: talking out of turn

surrender: allowing someone to speak before you

hook in: tying the person who surrendered back into the conversation

self-correct: monitoring one's behavior and making appropriate changes

Materials

poster board or butcher paper for brainstorming

any props needed for the role plays you create

Springboard

"I observe that you're all listening and are ready for CommunicationLab. In fact, last week we learned about listening. We also challenged you to teach your family about listening."

How did your family respond to your good listening?

Was anyone able to talk about talking when they couldn't give their full attention to listening?

Did anyone observe their family members trying to be better listeners?

How did that make you feel?

"Your good listening encourages me and makes me excited about teaching today's communication lesson. Today we're going to learn about turn taking."

Where are some places that we take turns?

Who are some people you take turns with?

What happens when someone doesn't wait for his turn?

How does it make you feel?

What do people say or do when you don't take your turn?

"Turn taking is important so people don't get angry and so everyone can be included, rather than excluded."

What does included *and* excluded *mean?*

"Okay, now that we know how important turn taking is, we're ready to plunge into the first Warm Up activity."

Warm Up

For Younger Students

Your younger students and self-contained classrooms will benefit from participating in the *Interruption* and *Maintain the Conversation* games as a whole class. Choose a student to join you in front of the class. After the activity, discuss the consequences of the teacher's interruptions with the entire group.

Interruption

Begin by having students pair up and have two-minute conversations. Have each pair decide who will be the primary talker and who will be the interrupter. The talker will talk on a selected topic, like her first memory of school or her favorite/worst teacher. The interrupter will interrupt the speaker at least three times.

Begin this activity and notice how the decibel level rises radically as people are interrupted—not to mention the rise in the frustration level. Now call "freeze!" Tell the interrupters to raise their hands. Ask if they had fun with this activity. Typically, these students will be laughing and will want to share what a great time they had. Now, ask the talkers to raise their hands. Ask them if they enjoyed the activity. This is a silly question since the answer is obvious, but you'll be making an important point. Comment on how interesting it is that the interrupters had such a good time while the speakers were frazzled.

Challenge your students to think about the following:

Why did the interrupters and speakers feel differently about this activity?

Talkers, what did the interruptions do to your speech?

Did you have to talk louder?

Could you keep track of what you were saying?

How did the interruptions make you feel?

Summarize this activity by sharing how interruptions not only aggravate us, but they also make it difficult for some people to communicate. Now your class is ready to participate in the next Warm Up activity which will help them learn how to take turns in a conversation.

Maintain the Conversation Game

Have your students remain in their original pairs to conduct another two-minute conversation on topics of their choice. This time, instruct the previous interrupter to enter the conversation at least three times without interrupting. Further explain that both communicators should observe how each speaker enters and exits the conversation successfully.

Following their two-minute conversations, call "freeze!" Explore your students' reactions to this activity with the following questions:

Why was the classroom quieter during this activity?

What else was different from the previous conversation with all the interruptions?

Did everyone have fun this time? Why?

How did not being interrupted affect both communicators' speech?

Brainstorming

On a poster board or butcher paper, list your students' observations of how people get in and out of conversations without interrupting. Your list might include the following:

To enter a conversation:

◆ Wait for a pause in the conversation.

◆ Answer if you're asked a question.

◆ When there is silence, comment on what the speaker has said.

◆ Say the speaker's name before you contribute to the conversation.

To exit a conversation:

◆ Summarize what the speaker said.

◆ Give the speaker feedback about what he said.

◆ Let the other communicator know you enjoyed the conversation.

This list of conversational turn-taking strategies will serve as an anchor for your students when they practice good turn taking following this communication lesson. Your students are now ready to practice these skills in role plays.

School, Friendship, & Home Role Plays

School

"Over-enthusiastic learners" is a generous way to describe the interrupters in our classrooms. Actually, many of the chief interrupters only talk out of turn because they're excited about what you're teaching, and they have something to contribute. Through role playing, your students will discover that interruptions cause the following:

◆ Interruptions sabotage others' learning.

◆ Interruptions make people frustrated or possibly angry at us.

◆ Interruptions deprive us of the positive feedback we were seeking in the first place.

Role Play 1
Consequences of Interrupting
Creating Role Plays

Create role plays that will teach your students the consequences of interrupting while the teacher is teaching. The classroom teacher will play the part of a student who is a constant interrupter. Select students to be the other classmates. Then, choose a student to play the role of the teacher.

Suggested Role Plays

While the student tries to teach the class, have the classroom teacher interrupt by doing one of the following:

◆ Continue to raise her hand furiously even after she's had a turn.

◆ Continue to shout out that she knows the answer.

- Whisper the answer to the student who was called on.
- Aggressively remind everyone else to wait their turn.

Assessing Role Plays

When the student who is playing the part of the teacher is thoroughly frustrated, call "freeze!" Begin brainstorming with these activating questions:

Who wasn't a good communicator?

What skill did this person forget to use?

What happened to all the other learners because of the interrupter's poor turn taking?

How did the student who was playing the role of the teacher feel?

What happened to the lesson because of poor turn taking?

Problem Solving

Invite your students to role play this situation again by using their turn-taking skills. Discuss how being a good turn taker can help you in school.

Role Play 2
Cutting In
Creating Role Plays

In the second role play, you'll teach your students how to problem solve when someone cuts in line. Create a role play where five students have to line up. The communication teacher will be one of the five students. Secretly instruct one of the students to budge in or cut right in front of the teacher. Have the teacher over-react by doing one the following:

Suggested Role Plays

- Start a fight.
- Whine to the teacher.
- Get others to gang up on the person who cut in line.
- Get angry and raise your voice.

Assessing Role Plays

Call "freeze" following the commotion from the teacher's over-reaction to the student cutting into the line. Brainstorm with your students to help them understand the following:

Who wasn't a good communicator?

What happened because of the way the teacher reacted to having someone cut in front of him?

How could the teacher have handled it differently?

Problem Solving

Select a group of students to role play this situation again. Challenge the students to use one of the suggestions for handling someone who cuts in front of them when they're in line.

For Older Students

By this point in the Lab, your older students will have the hang of the format, and they'll be ready to begin creating some of their own role plays without teacher participation.

Begin by asking students to recall times when they were interrupted in class, as well as times when someone cut in front of them. Invite them to recreate these situations so the rest of the class can see the consequences of poor communication.

91

Use the suggested *Assessing Role Plays* questions to debrief your students. Challenge these same students to role play the situation again using improved communication skills. Discuss the results of good turn taking.

Friendship

Being included by a peer empowers even the shyest of students to participate to their fullest. In fact, a recent study explored the role that peer relationships play in students' adjustments to school. The study concluded that being disliked by peers negatively colored a student's view of school, whereby the student developed higher levels of school avoidance and lower levels of school performance (Ladd, 1990). These role plays will teach your students the following:

◆ the consequences of excluding other people

◆ how to include others or get yourself included, even if a game has already begun

Role Play 1
Consequences of Exclusion
Creating Role Plays

Create a role play that will teach your students the consequences of people not wanting to include them in a game or on a team. You and the classroom teacher will play the roles of team captains. Enthusiastically begin choosing students to be on the individual teams. As you get down to fewer students to choose from, begin communicating in one of the following discouraging ways:

Suggested Role Plays

◆ Don't look as excited to have some people on your team as others.

◆ Use a disappointed tone of voice when you have to choose someone.

◆ Ask the coach if you have to choose anyone else.

Assessing Role Plays

Call "freeze" after the last student is chosen for a team. Since some of your students may feel sensitive following this role play, remind them that this is only a role play so we can learn what happens when we choose not to be good communicators. Then, begin debriefing with your students by asking the following:

Who wasn't a good communicator?

What happened because of your poor communication?

How did it make your students feel?

Which students will probably play better as a result of the way they were chosen for the teams?

Problem Solving

Invite two students to be the team captains of the teams and role play the situation again by using improved communication. Challenge these students to be good turn takers and to communicate encouragingly during their selection of fellow team members. Following their role play, ask the following:

How did the captain's communication make the team members feel?

How do you predict the players will play as a result of this communication?

For Older Students

Help students create a role play with the following activating question: "Can anyone think of a time when someone was chosen to be on a team, but you knew the team wasn't happy about having this person as a team member?"

Next, invite a group of students to re-create this situation in a role play so the class can learn the consequences of poor communication. Use the suggested *Assessing Role Plays* questions to debrief your students.

Challenge these same students to role play the situation again by using improved communication. Discuss the consequences of using good communicative behavior.

Role Play 2
Encouragement to Join a Group
Creating Role Plays

The second role play will teach your students how to notice when someone needs encouragement to join a group, as well as how to get themselves included.

Suggested Role Play

Create a role play where a game is getting started. One person is on the sideline watching, but is too shy to ask to join. Secretly instruct the role players not to extend an invitation to this shy classmate.

Assessing Role Plays

Call "freeze" following the action and begin debriefing by asking the following questions:

What was the problem?

How do we know that the student wanted to play but was too shy to ask?

What could the group have done differently to encourage and include this shy student?

What could the shy student have done to get included?

Problem Solving

Now that your students have some suggestions for handling the situation differently, challenge them to role play the situation again using some of the suggestions. Discuss the consequences of the communication suggestions they used.

Role Play 3
Excluding Carefully
Creating Role Plays

Once a game has already begun, it's difficult to get included. On the other hand, students need to learn that it isn't always appropriate to include someone after a game has begun. They need to learn how to communicate this without hurting other people's feelings.

Suggested Role Play

Create a role play where a game has already begun. Instruct a student to wander along and ask to join the group. The classroom teacher, who is playing the part of a student, will say in a rude tone of voice, "No, you can't play."

Assessing Role Plays

After the role play, call "freeze" and ask the following questions:

Who wasn't a good communicator?

How did it make the person who wanted to join feel?

What could have been done differently?

How could the person who wanted to join the game get himself included?

What could the person who wanted to join the game do while he's waiting to be included in the next game?

Problem Solving

Invite your students to role play this situation again using their suggestions. Remind them that it's difficult to include someone once a game has begun, but it's important to communicate in a kind way. You may suggest that they include the newcomer in the next game. Also suggest that there are ways newcomers can ask to be included that will encourage or discourage others from wanting them to join the group.

For Older Students

Help your students create a role play from the following activating question:

Can you remember a time when someone asked to join a game that had already begun?

Invite a group of students to role play what happened. Discuss whether the group could have included that person and how they let the person know that they couldn't join the group.

Then, have students role play the following options:

What are some other ways to let a person know that she can't be included because the game has already begun?

What can you do while you're waiting to be included?

Home

Parents, like teachers, have an overwhelming job trying to give all family members an equal amount of attention and to meet their individual needs. At times, it may feel like their family is coming at them from all directions, which they may be doing if family members haven't mastered the art of turn taking.

y meal time is the ideal place to observe turn taking at the peak of deterioration. Few families are exempt from an occasional meal where food is being passed in several directions, and little brother is trying to tell about his day at school with his mouth full, while his older sister is competing to ask for the car on Friday night.

I'm sure a few parents would love to call "freeze" and ask if their family could role play dinner again the right way! To eliminate the poor turn taking that goes on at home, have your students participate in the next two role plays that will teach them how to do the following:

◆ Observe before you communicate, so you don't interrupt.

◆ Take turns in a group situation.

◆ Surrender when two people begin talking at once.

◆ Hook the person who surrendered back into the conversation.

Role Play 1
Observing Before Communicating
Creating Role Plays

In the first role play, you'll teach your students to observe before they communicate so they don't interrupt. Choose a student to play the role of a parent who is busy with one of the following suggested scenarios. The classroom teacher can play the role of the child who enthusiastically charges into the room and begins telling all about his day.

Suggested Role Plays

◆ A parent is talking to a neighbor.

◆ A parent is taking a nap.

◆ A parent is paying bills.

Assessing Role Plays

After calling "freeze," debrief with your students by asking the following questions:

Who wasn't a good communicator?

What happened because you interrupted?

How did it make the parent feel?

How might the parent react because you didn't notice she was busy?

Problem Solving

Challenge a student to play the role of the child, but this time, the child should notice that the parent is busy and avoid interrupting. Debrief with your students to crystalize the consequences of good communication.

For Older Students

Help your students create a role play from the following activating question:

Have you ever tried to get your parents' attention and realized you interrupted them?

Invite a group of students to role play this scenario. Use the suggested debriefing questions to help your students understand the consequences of poor turn taking. Challenge this same group of students to role play this scene again by using improved turn-taking behavior. Discuss the consequences of good turn taking.

Role Play 2
Taking Turns in a Group
Creating Role Plays

In this second role play, your students will learn how to take a turn in a group.

Suggested Role Play

Create a dinner table scene with you and the classroom teacher playing the parts of siblings who are constantly interrupting everyone.

Assessing Role Plays

Following the role play, call "freeze" and debrief your students by asking the following questions:

Who wasn't a good communicator?

What happened because you were constantly interrupting?

How did that make the brothers, sisters, and parents feel?

How could the interrupters have communicated differently?

What can be done when two people begin talking at once?

Your students have given suggestions for what to do when two people begin talking at once. Follow up on their suggestions by teaching the concepts of *surrendering* and *hooking in*. First, ask your students if they know what *surrender* means. Then, ask a volunteer to begin talking at the same time as you so you can model surrendering. For example, you might say, "Mary Lynn, go ahead. What did you want to say?"

Remind Mary Lynn that she needs to hook you back into the conversation by saying, "Ms. Stone, what were you going to say?"

Problem Solving

Challenge your students to role play the situation again using their new communication tools of surrendering and hooking in.

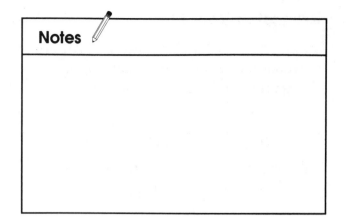

Communication Challenge

Challenge your students to go out of their way to include someone in their group activities. Further challenge your students to ask to be included in an activity with students who are less familiar to them.

Wrap Up

Help your students crystallize this lesson by commenting on how important turn taking is for school, home, and friendships.

Then help your students pinpoint where they need to work on their turn-taking behavior. Work with them to create a plan for improving their turn taking by asking the following questions:

In what ways do you think our class is already good at turn taking?

Where could we practice our turn-taking skills?

What can I do to remind you to take turns?

Classroom Carryover Activities

1. Monitor Turn Taking

This activity will help your students get an accurate reading of how often they participate verbally in your classroom. Prior to leading a group discussion in any content area, tell your students to take out a blank sheet of paper. Instruct them to mark down each time they contribute verbally to the class discussion so they can determine if they need to risk more verbally or if they need to give other people more opportunities to speak.

Following the discussion, have your students report their totals and make personal decisions about whether they need to take more or fewer turns in class discussions. Next time you lead a class discussion, activate your students' memories of their personal goals to monitor their turn taking.

2. Surrender and Hook In

It can be frustrating when everyone talks at once. Challenge your students to have a group discussion without raising their hands to gain a speaking turn. Primary teacher, Mary Stamos, uses this challenge as follows:

During her Writer's Circle, each student shares a story and then asks fellow classmates if they have any comments or questions. Students begin commenting and questioning by using their observations skills to exercise good turn taking instead of raising their hands. She reminds her students that if someone else begins talking at the same time, they can surrender. Mary also helps the person who gains the speaking turn to remember to hook the person surrendering back into the conversation.

In time, you'll no longer need to remind your students as they will automatically remember. When your students get this technique down, it will make for much more sane classroom conversations.

3. Include/Exclude

Students need practice asking to join a group. Select some simple and quick games, such as Twister, jacks, jump rope, or pick-up sticks. Have your students get into groups and play one of the games. Warn your students that when you ring a bell or call "freeze", all of the blue-eyed children should try to join another group.

Following this activity, brainstorm to pinpoint the difficulties that occur when trying to join an established group. Encourage your students to verbally problem solve to come up with solutions to these commonly occurring problems. You may repeat this activity on subsequent days so your students can gain the social skills that are necessary to get involved in and to organize group activities.

Parent Lab

1. Interruption/Maintain the Conversation

Play the *Interruption* game described on page 89 of this lesson. Debrief with family members following the game to identify interruptions, how the interruptions made the family feel, and what the interruptions did to their communication.

Proceed to the *Maintain the Conversation* game on page 89. Following the game, identify how family members effectively got in and out of the group's conversation.

Then, invite families to choose a time of day to play *Maintain the Conversation.* Ask that the family identify one positive method each family member can use to get into the conversation. For example, a parent might lean forward and ask, "Can I say something?"

Children who frequently interrupt or find it difficult to get into conversations usually find an "entry script" helpful. For example, a child could say, "Can I jump in?"

2. Think Out Loud

Think out loud with families about when and how they interrupt each other. A common time that children interrupt are when parents are on the telephone. Work together to create a way for all family members to "self-correct" or apologize when they interrupt. For example, a family member might say, "Excuse me for interrupting," or "Oops" (and then cover one's mouth and take a step back).

Then, create role plays so families can practice self-correcting these predictable interruptions. Remind parents to praise their child when she catches herself interrupting.

Dear Parents,

This week in CommunicationLab, we focused on turn taking. During the Lab, your child learned how to get in and out of a conversation without interrupting. Your child also learned how to self-correct (or apologize and wait his turn) when he accidentally interrupts. These turn-taking skills will prove useful to your child throughout his life. Practicing these skills as a family will reinforce what your child is learning in CommunicationLab.

Since meal time can be hectic when people don't take turns, we recommend that you invite your child to share the secrets for getting in and out of a conversation so your whole family can practice turn taking. At the end of the meal or over dessert, invite each family member to share her observations about the turn taking that occurred.

What made it easy or difficult for each person to get into a conversation? What can the rest of the family do to make it easy for everyone to get included? Challenge your family by asking each family member to think of one small thing he can do to improve his turn taking for the next family meal.

Taking turns will always be challenging. Let your child know when it's difficult for you to wait your turn. Since turn taking involves waiting, it's especially difficult for children. Adults can help children wait their turn by building up a trust so that the child will understand that she'll get a turn eventually, if she can just wait.

Sincerely,

Lesson 6: The Way We Communicate

Our choice of words is undeniably important when communicating. However, the *way* we communicate is remembered far longer than *what* we communicate. Think for a minute of a time when someone asked you to do something for him and you turned him down. Looking back, was it *what* he asked for or the *way* he asked for it that discouraged you from wanting to cooperate?

No doubt, the *way* we use vocal intonation and accompanying body language can either encourage or discourage peoples' cooperation. Many children are so focused on *what* they want that they forget to be aware of the *way* they communicate. Instead of getting the cooperation they were seeking, children frequently get into fights, make enemies, or receive parental and teacher reminders to change their attitudes.

In this CommunicationLab, you'll teach your students how to monitor their vocal inflection and body language so they can communicate in a way that will enlist others' cooperation. When designing role plays, recall situations in your class when students communicated with each other in ways that discouraged people. For instance, you might mention situations like the way someone asked to borrow something, how someone tried to get her pencil or seat back, or how a student asked for help or responded to a question.

Your students will have an opportunity to send *I messages* rather than *You messages* when they're upset with someone. When creating role plays, recall situations when your students were upset with another person's behavior and sent an accusing message like, "You always get to sit in that seat," rather than, "I feel disappointed that I never get to sit in that seat." It's the same message, only sent in a way that people can receive more easily since it's less aggressive.

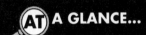

A GLANCE...

In this lesson on the way we communicate, you'll teach your students how to achieve the following:

◆ to understand how vocal intonation and body language can change the meaning of a message

◆ to communicate in a way that encourages others to cooperate

◆ to send *I Messages* rather than *You Messages*

◆ to send difficult messages in order to take care of themselves

◆ to take responsibility for their actions, rather than growing defensive or blaming other people

Your students will also have an opportunity to practice taking care of themselves by communicating their feelings and needs. Children, as well as adults, often find it difficult to risk asking for what they want, to send constructive criticism, or to tell someone how they really feel. For instance, if a student feels that an adult wasn't listening to her, she may find it difficult to tell the adult. If she chooses not to tell the adult, the listening situation between adult and child may never change, and the child may grow frustrated.

In this CommunicationLab, you and your students can brainstorm messages that are difficult to send, and then practice sending them in a way that will encourage others to listen. This Lab will also provide your students with an opportunity to take responsibility for their actions, rather than growing defensive and blaming others.

Vocabulary

encourage: communicating in a way that supports and promotes others' confidence

discourage: communicating in a way that causes someone to lose his self-confidence, spirit, and hope

taking care of yourself: communicate in a way that is true to one's values and feelings

mixed message: using words that communicate one message and body language that communicates another

clear message: using words and body language to communicate the same message

Materials

index cards

poster board or butcher paper for brainstorms

props necessary for the role plays you create

Springboard

Begin today's CommunicationLab by sending the following message three different ways. This activity will activate your students' awareness of how important voice and body language are when sending a message. Following your delivery of each message, wait for students to comment on your vocal inflections and body language.

"I'm really excited about teaching CommunicationLab."

first delivery	Act bored.
second delivery	Act puzzled and use a questioning vocal inflection.
third delivery	Act enthusiastic and energized.

Following this Springboard activity, tell your students that although you said the same message each time, you got three different responses. Ask your students the following:

Were my messages the same?

How were they different?

One of your students might use these exact words, "It was the way you communicated that was different!" Let your students know that they're right on target and that during today's CommunicationLab, they're going to learn that the way they communicate either encourages or discourages others. When saying the words *encourage* and *discourage,* use vocal inflection and body language to give your students some clues as to the meaning of these words. Then, ask whether anyone can tell you what *encourage* and *discourage* mean.

After this discussion, your students will be ready to move into the Warm Up activity.

Warm Up

Sending a Message Different Ways

In this activity, your students will send one message at least three different ways to discover the different results they can get because of the way they communicated. To tailor this activity for each classroom, have a discussion with the classroom teacher about the types of messages students send each other that often lead to confrontation and require intervention. Write each message on a separate index card. Some suggestions follow:

◆ That's my seat!

◆ I was next.

◆ Can I play?

◆ Be quiet.

◆ Stop it!

◆ Move over!

Invite two students to come to the front of the classroom. Give one of the students an index card with a message on it, and instruct her to send the message as many different ways as she can without changing the words. Tell the listener to react to each message according to the way the message was communicated. You may model with the classroom teacher so your students can see a repertoire of different vocal intonations, such as whining, demanding, questioning, bored, indifferent, or worried.

For Younger Students

You and the classroom teacher will send each other messages, and the students will observe and talk about why the listener responded the way she did.

Challenge your students to imitate various vocal inflections, such as demanding and whining, so they can use their voices and body language in different ways to get the results they want.

When your students are finished with this eye-opening Warm Up activity, they'll be eager to move into role plays to practice communicating in a way that will create a more cooperative and caring learning climate in your classroom.

School, Friendship, & Home Role Plays

School

Throughout their school day, students ask each other and adults for help, favors, and other personal requests. In this group of role plays, your students will discover that the way they communicate affects how people respond to them.

Role Play 1
Communicating to Discourage Cooperation
Creating Role Plays

To begin these role plays, brainstorm with the classroom teacher to recall common requests students make during the day that usually lead to confrontation and conflict. Next, invite a student to join you or the classroom teacher in a role play where the teacher plays the part of a student wanting something. The teacher will communicate in a way that discourages cooperation.

Suggested Role Plays

◆ Ask for a seat back.

◆ Ask to borrow the glue.

◆ Demand help with a difficult math problem.

Assessing Role Plays

Call "freeze" following the role play. Debrief with your students by asking the following questions:

Who wasn't a good communicator?

Why did you respond as you did?

Problem Solving

With your students, generate other ways you could have communicated that might have encouraged cooperation. Invite some of your students to role play these suggestions. Following each role play, discuss how the way they communicated encouraged cooperation.

For Older Students

Extend this role-playing section by asking the students to brainstorm other messages they send to each other in school that can create confrontation. For example, what do they say and do if they suspect someone took something that doesn't belong to him? Invite your students to role play these situations twice.

In the first role play, instruct them to communicate in a way that discourages cooperation. Following their role play, praise your students for knowing how to communicate in a way that aggravates others. Then, challenge these same students to communicate in ways that encourage cooperation and will be helpful rather than hurtful.

To assess these role plays with your students, explore the following:

Why is it difficult to remember to communicate with a helpful tone of voice?

How can we remind ourselves to monitor our tone of voice?

How can we remind each other to communicate in a helpful way?

How can teachers help you remember to communicate in a way that encourages cooperation?

Role Play 2
Responding with Respect
Creating Role Plays

In the next set of role plays, you'll teach your students how to respond in a way that is respectful, as well as how to take responsibility for their actions. Discuss with the classroom teacher situations when she asked a student a question and the student responded in a rude or defensive tone of voice. For example, students can grow defensive when a teacher reprimands them for not following a class rule. Under these circumstances, students are often frightened and end up communicating in a defensive, rude way. In these role plays, a teacher will play the part of the student who responds with a rude tone of voice, and a student will play the part of the teacher.

Suggested Role Plays

◆ The teacher asks a student if he left the cap off the glue.

◆ The teacher asks, "Who didn't return the stapler?"

◆ The teacher asks a disruptive student why she's talking when she should be listening.

Assessing Role Plays

Call "freeze" following the role play and debrief with your students using the following questions:

Who wasn't a good communicator?

Why do your students think you communicated the way you did?

Was it helpful? Why?

Problem Solving

Challenge a group of students to role play again by communicating in a way that is less defensive and rude. Discuss the consequences of this communication.

Friendship

Students often want to be included in a group activity or game but don't know how to communicate effectively to get themselves included. For example, some students simply stand on the sidelines hoping for an invitation to play, while others ask to play using poor timing or a rude tone of voice.

In this set of role plays, you'll teach your students how to communicate so people will want to include them.

Role Play 1
Discouraging Inclusion
Creating Role Plays

Have some of your students begin a game to demonstrate how the way people communicate can discourage others from wanting to include them. In this role play, you or the classroom teacher will play the part of a student who wants to get included in the game, but asks in an ineffective way.

Suggested Role Plays

◆ Demand to join a game.

◆ Tell the other game players that you can play better, and then ask to be included.

◆ Use a whining tone of voice when asking to be included.

◆ Threaten to tell the teacher if you're not included.

Assessing Role Plays

Who wasn't a good communicator?

What happened because of the way the student chose to communicate?

Problem Solving

Invite your students to role play these situations again by communicating in ways that encourage others to include the outsider into their group.

For Older Students

Extend this role-playing section by asking students to brainstorm ways people communicate that make others not want to include them. Invite your students to role play these situations. Following each role play, discuss why the group didn't want to include the outsider. On the chalkboard, list the behaviors that discouraged the group from including the outsider.

Challenge your students to problem solve more effective ways to communicate that may encourage friends to include them in the group. On the chalkboard, list the behaviors that encourage others to include their peers in a group.

Role Play 2
Expressing Feelings and Conveying Needs
Creating Role Plays

In this set of role plays, you'll help your students send difficult messages that express their feelings and convey their needs. You or the classroom teacher will play the part of a student who sends a difficult message in a way that makes someone feel understandably defensive. For example, the teacher playing the part of a student who wants to get included in a game might whine, "You never let me play with you!"

To create these role plays, recall situations when your students needed to take care of themselves by telling a friend how someone's behavior made them feel.

Suggested Role Plays

◆ Express how it felt when someone excluded you.

◆ Express how it felt when you heard someone talk behind your back.

◆ Express how it felt when someone embarrassed you in front of others.

Assessing Role Plays

Following the role play, discuss the following:

Who wasn't a good communicator?

How did it make the message receiver feel?

How could you have sent the same message in a different way?

Demonstrate how you can send a message that is easier to receive by changing it from a *You Message* to an *I Message*. For example, instead of saying, "You embarrassed me in front of my friends," you could say, "I felt embarrassed when

you ...ughed at me in front of my friends." Explore with your students the different feelings *You Messages* and *I Messages* produce. Which type of message is easier to receive? Why?

Problem Solving

Invite your students to role play sending various difficult messages. Suggest that they first send a *You message* and then an *I message*. Discuss which message is easier to receive.

Home

No doubt parents have consulted with you regarding their concerns about the attitudes of kids these days. Again, it's not so much what kids say, but the way they say things that aggravates and concerns parents. To help your students become aware of the way they communicate to their parents, create a series of role plays from the following brainstorm.

Role Play 1
Communicating for Cooperation
Creating Role Plays

Ask your students to recall favors they ask their parents, such as staying up late to watch TV or having a friend spend the night. Invite a group of students to role play these situations twice. In the first role play, instruct them to communicate in a way that would make their parents never want to cooperate. Praise them by saying something like, "You're so right. Your parents would never want to do that favor for you if you communicated that way!" Next, challenge them to role play the situation again by communicating in a way that might encourage their parents to cooperate.

Suggested Role Plays

◆ Ask a parent for a sleep-over party.

◆ Ask a parent for a family pet.

◆ Ask a parent for help with homework.

Assessing Role Plays

Following each version of the role play, discuss the subtle differences in the way your students sent the same message and the reactions they obtained.

How did they communicate?

What happened because of the way they communicated?

For Younger Students

You and the classroom teacher may need to role play so students can observe what happens when we demand or whine when requesting a favor. Use the suggested assessment questions to help your students discover why this kind of communication is fruitless.

Your students may then be ready to role play each situation again in a way that would encourage a parent's cooperation. However, some of your students may need you to initially role play the "right way" of communicating so they can use your suggestions as a model.

Role Play 2
Sending Mixed Messages
Creating Role Plays

In this set of role plays, you'll make your students aware of the way they respond to their parents when their parents ask them to help around the house.

To begin these role plays, have your students brainstorm to help them recall things their parents ask them to do around the house. For the first role play in this set, you or the classroom teacher will play the part of a child who communicates with a mixed message by using words that say one thing and body language that suggests another message. For example, your words might say, "Yeah, I'll take out the garbage," but your body language and tone of voice might be non-cooperative. Have a student play the part of the parent who has to receive this mixed message.

Suggested Role Plays

A child sends a mixed message when her parent asks her to do the following:

◆ take the garbage out

◆ help a younger sibling with her homework

◆ help rake the lawn

Assessing Role Plays

Following each role play, help your students discover the following:

Who wasn't a good communicator? Why?

What messages did the words send?

What messages did the body language send? (Explain that this is a mixed message—when our words say one thing and our body language says another.)

What happens when we send a mixed message?

How could the person have communicated differently?

Problem Solving

Invite your students to re-role play the situation by sending a clear message, where the words and body language match.

For Older Students

Extend this activity by brainstorming with students to recall other times when they responded to their parents' requests for help in a way that was aggravating. Again, have your students role play these situations twice, once by sending a mixed message and the second time by sending a clear message. Debrief with your students following each role play to pinpoint the difference sending a clear message can make.

Notes

Wrap Up

"Today we learned a lot about the importance of the way we communicate with one another. Sometimes, when we're mad, it's not easy to communicate in a way that encourages other people to cooperate. Let's brainstorm some reasons that make it difficult to communicate in a helpful way."

, let's brainstorm ways we can problem solve when it's difficult to communicate in a helpful way."

How can I remind you?

How can you remind yourselves?

How can we remind each other?

Help your students generate agreed upon signals or phrases they can use with each other to encourage improved communication.

Communication Challenge

Before giving your students their challenge, have them share their experiences with turn taking.

Did anyone catch himself interrupting?

Were you able to self-correct?

How do you think that made the other person feel?

Next, challenge your students to think of a person who makes it difficult to communicate with them because they easily make you angry. Then, challenge your students to communicate with this person in a helpful way the next time they have an opportunity.

Classroom Carryover Activities

1. Encourage Cooperation

Create a 20- to 30-minute period of time when your students can play various games in small groups. Suggestions for quick and simple games include pick-up sticks, jacks, jump rope, and ball-bouncing games.

Divide your class into groups and assign each group to a game. Warn your students that you're going to have one of the game players secretly try to sabotage the game. Each group's task is to try to communicate in a way that would encourage group cooperation rather than cause confrontation. Have some students rotate from game to game following each sabotage. Sabotages may include asking one of the players to whine, quit, cheat, be a poor sport, make fun of another player, or change the rules. (It's helpful to write these sabotages on individual index cards and then give them to the game players.)

After students have had several opportunities to send difficult messages in helpful ways, bring them back into a large group to debrief about game playing and communication.

2. Send Clear Messages

At the beginning of the day, remind your students about responding in a cooperative way when someone asks a favor. Warn them that you and some students whom you secretly select may ask them to do favors, like photocopying some papers, delivering something to the office, or straightening an area of the classroom.

Explain to your students that it's all right if they can't be helpful at that minute, just urge them to send clear messages. At the end of the day, bring your students together for a group discussion about that day's communication.

3. Ask for a Favor

Challenge your students to request favors from each other and from you throughout the day by using intonation and body language that encourages cooperation. At the end of the day, discuss your students' results. Were people happy to be helpful? Why do they think this was the case? If they couldn't help, how did they communicate this?

4. Self-Correct the Way You Communicate

At the beginning of the day, challenge your students to monitor the way they communicate with one another. Remind them that there may be times when they forget and hear themselves communicating in a hurtful, rather than helpful, way. Suggest to your students that on these occasions, they can self-correct by simply saying, "I don't like the way I communicated that, let me say it again."

Urge your students to monitor their communication and to self-correct throughout the day. At the end of the day, inquire to see if any of your students were able to self-correct. Or ask if they were able to catch themselves the first time and then self-correct by communicating with a positive tone of voice and good body language.

Parent Lab

1. Initiation

Have a discussion about tone of voice. Try to capture what it is about family members' communication that makes people want to be cooperative. Is it tone of voice, body language, word choice, timing, or all of these elements that create a positive communication environment?

Families frequently ask each other for help. Create a list of reasons family members ask each other for help. Next, create role plays and instruct family members to ask for help two different ways. The first time, have them ask in a way that would not encourage cooperation. Identify what it is about the tone of voice, body language, or timing that doesn't promote cooperation.

Then, role play again so family members can communicate in a way that encourages cooperation. Again, identify what it is about communication that makes people more apt to help.

Wrap up this activity by identifying when or where family members will be more aware of the way they're communicating, like when asking for a snack or for help with homework.

2. Tone of Voice

It can be difficult for people to monitor their tone of voice when frustrated, angry, or stressed. Work with the family to identify predictable stressful and/or frustrating moments. For example, the child might feel frustrated when writing a report on the computer.

Role play these situations and identify what people do to help the situation or how they make the situation worse. How do they communicate to themselves and each other?

Then, role play again so family members can practice communicating in a more positive way. Create a reminder signal or phrase so parents can cue their child to communicate in a more constructive manner when they become frustrated. For example, a parent can say, "Alexander, I know you're frustrated, but can you ask me for help in a nicer way?"

When families plan for these frustrating moments, children are often more responsive to making their communication more positive. Wrap up this exercise by choosing a time of day parents will use the reminder signal or phrase.

Dear Parents,

This week in CommunicationLab, your child learned that her tone of voice and body language can communicate an attitude that either encourages or discourages others to cooperate with her. We call this the *way* we communicate.

Now your child will know exactly what you mean when you remind her that you don't like the way she is communicating. Your child will also know how to change the way she says things so she can communicate with greater respect.

To help your child practice these new communication skills, ask him to show you different ways he can use his voice when requesting a favor. For instance, your child may ask if you could drive him to the store or to a friend's house. Following each of his attempts to get you to do the favor, tell your child how you would respond if he communicated using a whining, demanding, or angry tone of voice.

To further reinforce these good communication habits, seek opportunities to praise your child when she asks you for something or responds to you in a courteous and caring way.

Sincerely,

Lesson 7: Praise

"Good job!" "Way to go!" "That's it!" Teachers and parents are the first to encourage and support our children's efforts, kind actions, and accomplishments with a compliment or praise. Unfortunately, much of our praise is sent so generically, that exclaiming, "Terrific" often leaves children wondering what they did that was so terrific. It would be a fluke if they ever repeated the behavior.

In this CommunicationLab, your students will learn how to go to the source and communicate specific praise. That's right, go to the source. How often do we find ourselves praising someone behind his back? Children often will tell other people how much they appreciate a friend, teacher, or parent. Your students will learn how to go straight to the source so their friends, parents, and teachers can reap the benefits of the praise.

When designing role plays, recall positive behaviors you want your students to be aware of, such as listening, sharing, compromising, and exercising patience. Once you have identified these positive behaviors through role playing, you can teach your students how to acknowledge these qualities in their peers, parents, and teachers and how to send specific praise to the source!

In order to encourage people to continue praising us, we must receive their praise. Certainly we can all remember a time when we complimented someone and he didn't accept our praise. You may have told someone how much you liked her outfit, and she responded, "This old rag?" In other words, she indirectly told you that you have bad taste in fashion. Now, what are the chances of you praising this person again in the near future? Slim at best!

The important point is that children with low self-esteem who would benefit the most from praise may be blatantly or subtly dis-couraging others from praising them because they aren't accepting

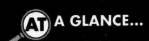

AT A GLANCE...

In this lesson on praise, you'll teach your students how to achieve the following:

- become aware of the power of praise
- send specific, sincere praise
- receive praise
- seek out reasons to praise peers, parents, and teachers
- feel proud about their own efforts, kind actions, and accomplishments

the praise. It could be that some children are overwhelmed or embarrassed by praise, so they change the subject, praise back, or simply look away.

This CommunicationLab will teach your students how to receive praise so they can encourage others to continue praising them. We want to help create a learning and home environment where people seek out the good in others, as well as become more aware of their own valuable contributions. People often tend to be hard on themselves and others. Think about a day when you received a generous amount of praise and little criticism. What do you tend to remember and dwell on at the end of the day? Naturally, most people dwell on the criticism because we're constantly striving to improve.

Our children learn new things every day, and they experience successes and failures. You can assume that your students have high expectations for themselves. Therefore, like us, they'll dwell on what went wrong during the day rather than what went right. In this lesson, you'll help your students learn to be generous with praise to themselves and to others.

Vocabulary

specific: sending praise that communicates exactly what one likes

sincere: sending honest praise

receive: acknowledging praise that is sent to you

lift up: communicating a message that lifts up the receiver's spirit

Materials

two hula hoops (You may substitute a jump rope or ball.)

wig (optional)

chalkboard

props necessary for role plays you create

Springboard

Immediately upon starting CommunicationLab, choose any four students in the class and praise them. Give a warm smile and sincere, but generic praise to two of the students. For example, you might say, "Good job, Mark!" Then send sincere, specific praise to the other two students such as, "Joan, I appreciate your attention!"

Following this praise activity, call "freeze!" Ask the students to whom you sent the generic praise what they did that was so good. Some students may guess something like, they were listening or paying attention. Ask them if they're sure that's what they did that was good. They'll have to say "No" because you weren't specific in your praise. Then ask them if they could repeat the behavior. With puzzled faces, again they'll have to say "No."

Repeat the same process with the two students who received specific praise. Explain that because these students received specific praise, they could repeat that good behavior again if they wished. Ask if anyone knows what *specific* means. Following your students' understanding of this concept, summarize as follows: "Today in CommunicationLab, we're going to learn how to send specific praise so our friends, teachers, and parents know what they are doing that we like. Let's discover some other important things about praise. I need a volunteer to praise me about my outfit."

Have a student praise you about your outfit, but don't receive the praise. You may choose to ignore it altogether, change the subject, or tell her that you hate the outfit. Discuss the student's reaction to your not receiving her praise. Would she be encouraged to praise you again? Why? Explain that praise not only has to be specific, but it also must be received.

Warm Up

The Power of Praise

Invite two volunteers to come to the front of the classroom to participate in a hula hoop activity. (If your school doesn't own hula hoops, substitute jump ropes or balls.) Lavish encouragement and praise on the first student who volunteers, while merely handing the hula hoop to the second volunteer. Next tell them to twirl the hula hoops around them as many times as they can. While the students are struggling with the hoops, give the first student the majority of your attention, while offering a few token "good jobs" to the second student. Nearly always you'll find that the second student grows discouraged and quits. This is the perfect time to call "freeze!"

Ask your students to discuss what they observed. Debrief with them regarding the power of positive attention and praise. Explain that you weren't being mean to the second student, but you just didn't communicate in a way that showed you cared. Remind your students that praise can encourage people to do their best. Explain that in CommunicationLab, your students will learn to lift up themselves and others by sending praise.

Sincere Praise

To help your students learn the importance of sending sincere praise, role play the following scenario with the classroom teacher. Have the classroom teacher wear a silly wig (or put her hair in an unusual style) and give her praise with words, but "funny looks" with your body language. After it seems clear to your students that you're sending insincere praise, call

"freeze." Discuss the importance of sending sincere praise.

Go to the Source

To help your students understand the importance of going to the source (by communicating directly with the person who deserves the praise), role play the following scenario with the classroom teacher.

Invite a student to join you and the classroom teacher for this role play. Begin by having a three-way conversation. Have the student leave shortly so only the two of you are left. After the student leaves the conversation, tell the classroom teacher how wonderful you think the student is at writing creative stories. Call "freeze" following this scenario.

Debrief with your students to help them discover that the student will never benefit from this praise because he didn't hear it first hand. Remind your students to go to the source when they have something nice to say.

School, Friendship, & Home Role Plays

School

Your students are continually interacting with each other, their parents, and teachers in ways that deserve praise. In this set of role plays, your students will learn how to send specific praise, as well as how to receive praise.

Creating Role Plays

Before beginning these role plays, brainstorm with the classroom teacher to generate a list of things that her students do that are praise-worthy. Ask for volunteers to be in a role play while you or the classroom teacher narrate the action. For example, you might say, "The students were lining up for a drink of water, and Matthew remembered to go to the end of the line rather than take cuts in line." See if the other students remember to send specific praise and whether the praise is accepted.

Suggested Role Plays

◆ Students line up for a drink, and someone begins to cut in, but then they remember to go to the end of the line.

◆ A student returns something she found that doesn't belong to her.

◆ Someone waits patiently for a turn.

◆ Someone saves a seat for a friend.

◆ Students include a newcomer in their game.

Assessing Role Plays

After the action, call "freeze" and ask your students the following:

Did anyone deserve to be praised?

Was the praise sent specifically?

Was the praise received?

Problem Solving

If necessary, invite your students to role play these situations again, only this time send specific praise. When a student merely says, "Thank you," to someone who doesn't cut in front of them, the communication teacher can remind them to send specific praise by saying, "What are you thanking them for? Try saying, 'Thank you for not cutting in front of me.'"

Following your students' successful re-role play of this scenario, ask the praise-giver the following:

Would you be encouraged to praise this student again? Why?

the praise-receiver the following:

Were you encouraged to go to the end of the line rather than cut in? Why?

Create a few more role plays so students can gain additional practice sending and receiving specific praise. You'll be ready to progress to the next set of role plays when you no longer need to stop and remind your students to be more specific with their praise.

For Older Students

To design role plays, begin with the following brainstorm:

What things do your parents, teachers, and friends do that are praiseworthy? (List on the chalkboard.)

Next, have your students recreate these situations in role plays, remembering to send and receive specific praise. Use the suggested *Assessing Role Plays* questions to debrief with your students.

Friendship

Creating Role Plays

In this set of role plays, you'll teach your students the importance of receiving praise. You or the classroom teacher will play the role of a student who doesn't receive praise by denying the praise, acting embarrassed, or ignoring the praise altogether.

Suggested Role Plays

◆ A fellow student praises your new haircut.

◆ A friend admires how good you are at playing the flute.

◆ A neighbor praises your ability to ride a skateboard smoothly.

Assessing Role Plays

Call "freeze" following the role play and debrief with your students with the following questions:

Was the praise received?

How do you think that made the person sending the praise feel?

Does that encourage the person to send praise again?

Problem Solving

Invite your students to role play these situations again so they can practice receiving praise. Discuss how receiving the praise made the person sending the praise feel.

For Older Students

To help your students create a role play which will allow them to practice receiving praise, ask the following activating question:

Have you ever praised someone when they didn't receive it?

Invite students to illustrate this scenario in a role play. Following their role play, debrief with your students using the suggested *Assessing Role Plays* questions. Then, challenge your students to role play the situation again by receiving the praise.

Home

This set of role plays will give your students opportunities to practice praising their parents. During their role play, remind your students to send their parents specific praise.

Creating Role Plays

Design role plays to give your students opportunities to see their parents performing praise-worthy actions.

Suggested Role Plays

The parent will do the following for his child:

◆ help her with her homework

◆ prepare a favorite meal

◆ listen to his story with interest

◆ take care of her when she is sick

Assessing Role Plays

Following the action, call "freeze" and explore the following with your class:

Did the parent deserve praise?

Was the praise received?

Was the praise sent specifically?

If not, how could it have been sent more specifically?

How do you think praising makes your parents feel?

Problem Solving

If necessary, invite this group of students to role play the situation again, this time sending specific praise. Create additional role plays so other students can have opportunities to send their parents specific praise.

For Older Students

Create role plays from the following brainstorm:

What do my parents do that I wish they did more often?

List these ideas on the chalkboard so your students can use them to design their own role plays. Challenge your students to role play sending their parents the specific praise they deserve. Use the suggested *Assessing Role Plays* questions to debrief with your students.

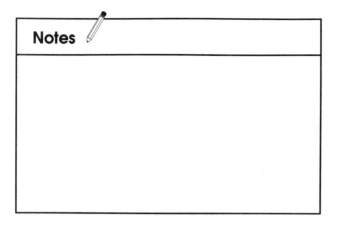

Notes

Wrap Up

"Today you were terrific in CommunicationLab! Did I send you specific praise? Let's brainstorm to recall all the things you did that were terrific, so I can send you specific praise." After you send more specific praise, make sure your class receives the praise so you can comment on how they received it.

What else did you learn about praise?

What are some reasons to praise friends? Teachers? Parents?

How did receiving praise make you feel?

Conclude the Wrap Up by reminding your students that praise makes us feel good inside. Further suggest that even if we don't receive praise from our friends, teachers, or parents, we can know inside ourselves that we can be proud of our actions. Brainstorm with your students to discover reasons they are proud of themselves. Examples might include being helpful to a younger sibling when the student has better things to do, or sticking with homework even when it's difficult.

Communication Challenge

Have your students talk about the communication challenge from the previous week where they had to communicate in an encouraging way with someone they have had a hard time getting along with.

Then, explain the new communication challenge to your students. Have them give three specific praises a day. One praise should go to a friend, one to a teacher, and one to someone they live with. Remind your students to remember the three people's reactions when given the praise. The following questions might help your students:

How did the praise make the people feel?

Did they repeat the behavior after you praised them?

Did they receive the praise?

If they didn't receive the praise, how did that make you feel?

Classroom Carryover Activities

1. **The Praise Whip**

Many of your students will need a lot of practice sending and receiving praise. The "Praise Whip," which I learned from primary teacher Judy Pringle, is a fun way to put praise into each of your school days.

At the end of the school day, gather your students into a circle so everyone can see each other. One at a time, everyone in your class will send and receive some uplifting praise. Begin the Praise Whip by turning to the person on your left and sending a specific praise. Her job is to receive the praise with either a smile or a "thank you" and then to send a praise to the next person in the circle. This activity is not only a great way to give your students practice sending and receiving praise, but it will also end everyone's day on a uplifting note!

2. **Proud Time Whip**

Special Ed teachers Paula Eash and Ed Phipps have created a "Proud Time Whip" at the end of their day. In this activity, each person in the circle has an opportunity to express what she did that day in school of which she is proud. If a student seems to be having a hard time recalling something to be proud of, ask him if he needs help. If the student would like help, his classmates can offer suggestions of things they have observed that they think their friend can be proud of.

3. **Caught Ya!**

At the beginning of the school day, challenge your students to see how many times they can catch someone doing something good and then send a specific praise. Bring your students together at the end of the day to debrief on all of the positive communication that echoed through your classroom that day. Further challenge them to try to catch their siblings and parents doing things that are praiseworthy.

4. **Team Work**

Often, academic projects require that you group your students. During one of these group projects, invite your students to notice when their classmates contribute to the group in helpful ways. Encourage them to send each other specific praises. Come together as a class to discuss this team-building activity.

119

Parent Lab

1. Sending Praise

Have family members divide into pairs. Ask each person to think of two reasons she appreciates her partner. Give family members opportunities to give and receive praise. Remind the praise-givers to be specific and sincere. You might need to demonstrate the qualities of effective praise giving. Cue the receiver of the praise to maintain eye contact and say "thank you."

Debrief following this exercise to pinpoint what makes it easy/difficult to give and receive praise. Clarify the importance of *not* evaluating praise, but rather accepting praise with a smile or thank you.

Wrap up this activity by asking family members how often they will send praise on a daily basis. Remind and demonstrate the usefulness of nonverbal praises, such as a smile or a pat on the back.

2. Identifying Communication Behaviors

Think out loud with each family member and identify a communication habit or behavior he'd like to improve. Challenge family members to praise one another for actively working on communication. For example, if the child wants to improve his eye contact while talking, his family would want to notice when he is using increased eye contact.

During this communication exercise, ask family members to:

◆ choose a communication habit to improve

◆ decide when and/or where they'll actively practice the new behavior

◆ pinpoint how they would like family members to praise them for using the new behavior

◆ decide how they will respond to the praise

Dear Parents,

This week in CommunicationLab, your child not only learned the importance of praise, but he also learned how to send and receive specific praise. Ask your child to share some of the things he learned about sending and receiving praise.

Your child learned that praise needs to be specific. For example, rather than saying, "Good job," we can communicate more specifically by saying, "What a nice job you did making your bed this morning." Specific praise is more powerful because it lets a person know exactly what was done that was appreciated. Your child also learned to receive praise with a smile or a simple "thank you" rather than ignore it.

Your family can brainstorm ways to incorporate more praise into your daily lives. You might like to participate in a family "Praise Whip" or "Proud Time Whip" activity. Your child's classroom teacher will be using these praising activities in her classroom and can give you the instructions so your family can enjoy these self-esteem building activities.

However you choose to enrich your child's lesson on praise, you'll help contribute to her increased self-esteem and reinforce what we have practiced in CommunicationLab.

Sincerely,

Lesson 8:
Criticism

Just like praise, criticism is an important part of communication in that it lets people know how they're doing. Although teachers and parents seek to reinforce children's praiseworthy efforts, kindness, and accomplishments, it's also important to give children constructive criticism. The challenge comes in how we send and receive criticism.

Criticism can be as difficult for people to send as to receive since many people don't want to have their feelings hurt, nor do they want to hurt the feelings of others. In this communication lesson, your students will learn how to send criticism to their peers, teachers, and parents in a helpful, constructive way. Likewise, they'll learn how to view criticism as helpful and will be able to receive criticism to help themselves make improvements. This skill will be especially useful for students who are struggling academically or socially since they tend to receive a higher percentage of criticism than other students.

Regardless of how hard we try, sometimes we find ourselves sending destructive criticism. In this lesson, students will learn how to self-correct when they recognize that they have sent hurtful criticism. Your students will also develop coping strategies to help them deal with direct put-downs. Criticism is usually remembered far longer than praise, so let's teach our students how to get criticism to work for them!

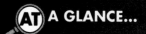

A GLANCE...

In this lesson on criticism, you'll teach your students how to:

◆ become aware of the usefulness of criticism

◆ send constructive, helpful criticism

◆ receive criticism and use it to make self-improvements

◆ self-correct when they catch themselves sending hurtful criticism

◆ provide assistance to a peer without taking over

◆ develop strategies to cope with destructive, hurtful criticism

Vocabulary

helpful criticism: sending criticism with the intent to help another person make improvements

hurtful criticism: sending criticism with the intent to put down another person

Materials

chalkboard

poster board or butcher paper

props necessary for role plays you create

Springboard

"You all look uplifted from last week's lesson on praise."

Were you able to send three specific praises a day? Tell me about some of the praises.

How do you think it made people feel?

Did they receive your praise?

How did it make you feel?

"This week in CommunicationLab, we're going to learn how to send and receive criticism."

Can anyone tell me what criticism means?

Does anyone like to receive criticism? Why?

Warm Up

During today's communication Warm Up Activity, you and the classroom teacher will role play to demonstrate various ways your students can send constructive criticism.

Can Do Criticism

When we send criticism for the first time, we can give others the benefit of the doubt by assuming that they didn't have the necessary information to be successful. Therefore, when sending criticism on these occasions, we can tell a person what they *can do* rather than what they *should have done.*

In the first role play, you and the classroom teacher will be modeling this "can do," rather than "should have done," criticism technique.

two students to come to the front of the room and sit at desks that face their classmates. Instruct the two students to use books and papers to mess up the tops of their desk so you can criticize them. Then, approach the first student with a curt voice and scold, "You should have a clean desk." Approach the second student with a firm, but constructive tone of voice and inform him, "Put your books on the left corner of your desk because I expect your desk to be straightened for class."

Call "freeze" and begin debriefing with your students to ask what they noticed about your contrasting body language, tone of voice, and choice of words. Discuss that with the second student, you gave a clear message of what is expected, rather than telling the student what they should have done. Clarify that when we send criticism, we need to give people information about what they can do, not what they should have done. Until now, they may not have known any differently.

For Older Students
3 + and a Wish

In this role play, you'll provide your students with another technique for sending constructive criticism. I've found this technique to be useful in my own life as well. Choose a student to join the classroom teacher. The classroom teacher will tell the student three specific things he's doing successfully and one thing she wants him to improve upon. For example, "I appreciate that your desk is always neat, that you're prepared for class, that you're attentive, AND, I wish you would get to school on time."

Following this role play, debrief with your students to help them become aware of the three pluses or praises and your wish or criticism. Point out that it's 3+'s AND a wish, not 3+'s BUT a wish. Remind them that once they say "but," they erase all the pluses before the wish! Then your students will have the tools they need to practice sending criticism through role playing.

School, Friendship, & Home Role Plays

School

Role Play 1
Sending Criticism
Creating Role Plays

Criticism is an appropriate part of an academic day since students naturally need suggestions on how they can improve their efforts. In these role plays, your students will learn how to send and receive criticism.

First, you and the classroom teacher will recall criticism you have observed your students sending each other. (See the Suggested Role Plays for additional ideas.) Invite a student to role play with the classroom teacher. As the student role plays sending criticism, the teacher will send hurtful, destructive criticism back to him (like a dirty look or a negative tone of voice) in order to motivate the student to be more careful about the kind of criticism he sends.

Suggested Role Plays

◆ Someone is distracting you by tapping a pencil on her desk.

◆ Someone is standing too close to you.

◆ Someone has taken too long a turn on the computer.

Assessing Role Plays

Following your first role play, call "freeze" and think aloud with your students about the following:

Who wasn't a good communicator? Why?

Was the criticism helpful or hurtful?

How did it make the receiver and sender feel?

Was it difficult to receive the criticism? Why?

How could the criticism have been sent differently?

Problem Solving

Challenge your students to role play again by sending criticism in a more helpful, constructive way. Create one or two more role plays where your students will send constructive criticism. Following each of these role plays, discuss how the criticism was sent and received.

For Older Students

Help students create their own meaningful role plays by writing the following brainstorm on the chalkboard:

What are some of the reasons I send criticism to my friends?

List each suggestion on the chalkboard. Invite students to role play sending one of the criticisms in a destructive, hurtful way. Then, use the suggested *Assessing Role Plays* questions to debrief your students. Finally, challenge your students to role play this scenario again by sending constructive criticism. Discuss the results they received because of improved communication.

Role Play 2
Receiving Criticism
Creating Role Plays

Recall occasions when your students have grown defensive because they were the recipients of criticism. (See the Role Play Suggestions for additional ideas.) You and the classroom teacher will role play growing defensive when someone sends you criticism.

Suggested Role Plays

◆ Blame someone else.

◆ Cry, whine, or throw a tantrum.

◆ Reciprocate the criticism.

Assessing Role Plays

Think aloud with your students and explore why we get defensive and angry when we're criticized.

What happened when your students were criticized?

Was this reaction helpful? Why?

Why do people criticize?

What can we do when we hear criticism?

How can we use criticism for our own self-improvement?

Following this group discussion, you and the classroom teacher will role play how to receive criticism without growing defensive.

Problem Solving

After your students observe you and the classroom teacher using criticism to help you make self-improvements, invite students to experience receiving criticism so they can practice.

For Older Students

Help students create their own meaningful role plays by writing the following brainstorm on the chalkboard:

What kind of criticism is difficult to receive from friends, parents, and teachers?

From your students' suggestions, have students role play growing defensive and angry when they hear constructive criticism.

Following their role play, think aloud with your students to explore the following:

Why do we get defensive?

Is being defensive helpful?

What might we do to help us handle criticism?

Problem Solving

Ask your students to role play each situation again to discover new and more helpful ways to receive criticism. Some of your students may initially require your help to model some constructive ways to receive criticism, such as listening attentively; asking the sender for more information on how you can improve; or thanking the sender for the helpful, constructive criticism.

To conclude these role plays, remind your students that few people enjoy hearing criticism, but it helps if we remind ourselves that the criticism was only sent to give us suggestions on ways we can make self-improvements.

Friendship

In the next group of role plays, you'll help your students recognize various types of hurtful criticism and explore methods to help them manage such criticism. Then, they'll have opportunities to self-correct when they send destructive criticism. To transition into this section of today's Lab, let your students know that they're going to learn how to receive hurtful criticism since, unfortunately, people don't always remember to be good communicators.

Creating Role Plays

Begin by writing the following brainstorm on a poster board or butcher paper that you'll leave in the classroom:

Ways to Respond to Hurtful Criticism

Next, ask a student to send the classroom teacher (who is playing the role of a classmate) hurtful criticism. This will provide the teacher with an opportunity to model various ways to respond and cope with destructive criticism. Your students may have some additional suggestions of their own, so give students an opportunity to share their suggestions by inviting them to role play. List all the coping strategies your class discovers (as illustrated below).

Ways to Respond to Hurtful Criticism

Ignore it.

Change the subject.

Walk away.

Compliment the criticizer.

Act shocked.

In a calm voice, tell the person how it made you feel.

Use a sense of humor, such as thanking them for the compliment.

Tell the teacher or an adult if it becomes too overwhelming.

Role Play 1
Strategies for Handling Destructive Criticism
Creating Role Plays

After your students have discovered numerous ways to handle destructive criticism, provide them with an opportunity to test some of these suggestions. This activity will give your students coping strategies they can use throughout their lives.

Problem Solving

For Younger Students

Select a student to receive hurtful criticism from either you or the classroom teacher. When you send hurtful criticism to this student, have him use one of the suggested strategies for handling destructive criticism. Challenge the rest of the class to pinpoint which strategy was used. Discuss which strategies your students feel they could use when they receive hurtful criticism.

For Older Students

Your students can send each other destructive criticism without your involvement. Have them either come up with role plays of their own or provide them with one of the following suggested role plays. Challenge your students to use one of the provided strategies to handle hurtful criticism. Discuss which strategies your students think they could really use when they receive hurtful criticism.

Suggested Role Plays

◆ Send a dirty look when someone steps on your foot.

◆ Yell at someone for being too loud.

◆ Laugh at someone when they make a mistake.

◆ Tell the person their outfit looks silly.

Assessing Role Plays

Following each role play, discuss how each person responded to the hurtful criticism.

Which technique did they use to handle the hurtful criticism?

Was it helpful? Why?

Role Play 2
Self-Correcting
Creating Role Plays

Suggest to your students that sometimes we hear ourselves sending criticism in hurtful ways. Provide them with an opportunity to observe you self-correct when you catch yourself being a poor communicator. In a role play situation, send destructive criticism to the classroom teacher and then self-correct.

Suggested Role Plays

◆ Someone criticizes, "Can't you get anything right?"

◆ Someone laughs at a peer's mistake.

◆ Someone tells a peer her idea is dumb.

Assessing Role Plays

Call "freeze" following the role play and debrief with your students using the following questions:

What was hurtful about our communication?

How do we know when we have been hurtful?

How did we self-correct?

Why do you think it's important to self-correct?

Problem Solving

Provide opportunities for your students to self-correct when they catch themselves sending hurtful criticism. Ask your students to recall times when they accidentally sent hurtful criticism. Next, have them role play one of the situations, demonstrating how to self-correct. If your students get stumped and can't recall a time when they sent hurtful criticism, provide them with some practical suggestions. Following their success with self-correcting, discuss how it made everyone involved in the interaction feel.

Role Play 3
Providing Help to a Classmate
Creating Role Plays

In this set of role plays, you'll teach your students how to provide help to one another instead of taking over. Begin by brainstorming all the situations in which they might need their friends' help. (List these ideas on the chalkboard.) Next, have the classroom teacher play the part of a student who takes over for another student, rather than demonstrating or telling the friend how to do something for himself.

Suggested Role Plays

◆ When a student is struggling to cut out a shape, take the paper away from her and complete it.

◆ When a student is having a difficult time solving a math problem, solve it for him.

Assessing Role Plays

Following this role play, think aloud with your students to help them realize how taking over for someone is not as helpful as giving the person the tools she needs to accomplish tasks for herself. Then, role play the situation again with the classroom teacher by modeling how to ask a person if she wants help. You might demonstrate for the person or verbally coach her so she can be successful on her own!

Problem Solving

Provide your students with an opportunity to act in role plays where someone needs help. Create these role plays from the previous brainstorm about things your students need help with from their friends. Encourage your students to ask if their friend needs help, and then either demonstrate or verbally coach their friend through the process.

Home

It can be very threatening for a child to send an adult criticism, and yet children have a right to voice their opinions. In the next role plays, you'll provide your students with opportunities to grow more confident in sending constructive criticism to their parents and other adults.

Creating Role Plays

List your students' ideas for this brainstorm on the chalkboard:

What are some reasons I criticize my parents?

After receiving their suggestions, invite one of your students to be the parent so you can model sending helpful criticism. During these role plays, remind your students how to talk about talking in order to soften the pain of the difficult message. For instance, you might say to a parent, "This is difficult for me to say because I love you, and I don't want to hurt your feelings, but I feel sad when I come home from school and you don't have time to listen to me or play with me."

Suggested Role Plays

◆ A parent never asks you how your day was.

◆ A parent forgot to follow through on a promise.

◆ A parent constantly interrupts.

Assessing Role Plays

After you model how to send a parent constructive criticism, discuss the students' reactions to your communication.

Would your parent be able to receive this kind of criticism?

Does anyone have any additional suggestions for sending a parent criticism?

Problem Solving

From your students' previous brainstorm (What are some reasons I criticize my parents?), create role plays so students can practice sending these difficult messages. Discuss what makes criticism easier to send and to receive.

For Younger Students

Have different students play the role of the child while you play the role of the parent. Challenge them to send a difficult message to their parent.

For Older Students

Older students can play the roles of both parent and child while practicing sending difficult messages.

Notes

Wrap Up

"Today we learned that criticism is difficult to send and to receive when we're aware of other people's feelings."

What are some things you can do to send criticism in a helpful way?

What are some strategies you can use if someone sends you hurtful criticism?

Then, praise how considerate your students are of each other's feelings. Ask your students for some suggestions on how you might remind them to send helpful, rather than hurtful, criticism. When you hear them forgetting to use helpful criticism, remind them with words or the agreed upon signal.

Communication Challenge

Challenge your students to send you and the classroom teacher constructive criticism about your teaching. Remind them to observe how you receive their criticism.

Then, ask your students if any of them would like you to send helpful criticism to them this week. Recruit volunteers to receive constructive criticism. Observe how they receive the criticism.

Classroom Carryover Activities

1. Sending and Receiving Criticism

At the beginning of a school day, challenge your students to be aware of how they're sending and receiving criticism. Invite them to notice when they send criticism and to ask the receiver if he felt it was sent in a helpful way. When any of your students receive criticism, invite them to comment to the sender about the way the criticism was sent.

Bring your students together at the end of the day to discuss their experiences and to brainstorm to determine how they could further improve their skills in sending and receiving criticism.

2. On the Home Front

Encourage your students to participate in the above activity with their families so criticism can be sent in a helpful way at home. Have your students share their observations the next morning.

3. Hooray for Me

This activity will teach your students how to give themselves constructive criticism. Just like in the *Praise Whip,* gather your students into a circle facing each other. Begin the activity by sharing something that you said or did that you'd like to do differently the next time. Encourage each student to think of one thing she could improve upon and share it with the group. At the end of the activity, praise your students for their honesty and ability to know exactly what they need to work on. Find out if there is any way you or their classmates can help them make these self-improvements.

Parent Lab

1. What Is Criticism?

Have a discussion about what criticism is. How is it used within the family? Is it helpful? Have family members look at who they criticize most in the family. How do they communicate this criticism?

Next, challenge family members to think of one way they could improve how they communicate criticism. For example, they might change their tone of voice or improve their timing.

Then, ask family members to choose one person in the family who they will communicate criticism to more carefully. Help family members set up a time during the week so they can communicate any positive changes in the way they're communicating criticism.

2. Receiving Criticism

The ability to receive constructive criticism is important. Discuss and/or demonstrate the difference between receiving criticism in a defensive and nondefensive manner.

Have family members share how it feels when they receive criticism. Does anyone in the family have an easier time with this than others? If so, what does this person do when receiving criticism? Is his technique something other family members could use?

Have family members choose a person within the family who they'll practice receiving criticism from in a less defensive way.

Help family members create a time during the week to give each other positive feedback on how family members are receiving criticism. Remind them that criticism is much easier to hear when given by a person who has previously sent a lot of praise.

Dear Parents,

No doubt following last week's CommunicationLab, your home is echoing with family members communicating praise to one another! This week, your child learned about an equally important communication tool — sending and receiving constructive criticism. Many people feel that criticism is as difficult to send as it is to receive.

During CommunicationLab, your child learned new ways to send criticism. Ask your child to teach you about "can do" criticism rather than "should have done" criticism. Your child can also share the new strategies for receiving criticism that we learned. Your child can teach you about accepting criticism by listening, asking for more information, and thanking the person who gave the criticism for being helpful.

If your family is interested in practicing sending and receiving criticism, you may wish to choose a special time during the week when each family member can share one thing he personally wants to improve upon and one thing which he wishes a family member would work on. Family activities like these help build everyone's trust and confidence.

Sincerely,

Lesson 9: Success and Failure

Your students will experience success and failure throughout their lives. In this communication lesson, you and the classroom teacher will teach your students the following:

◆ how to communicate with themselves and with others when experiencing success and failure

◆ how to manage their successes and failures

These communication skills are essential since external and internal communication are critical elements in encouraging and supporting future success.

Reflect for a moment on how your students communicate to someone when that person succeeds. Do you see a lot of put-downs or jealous challenging such as, "You think that's good? Watch this!" And, how do your students communicate about their own successes? Do they boast or act embarrassed? How much nicer and supportive it would be if your students knew how to communicate pride for themselves and for others when success is experienced. Likewise, wouldn't it be remarkable if your students could begin to learn from others' successes and to offer helpful suggestions from their own successful experiences? In this communication lesson, your students will have an opportunity to learn how to communicate in a way that fosters pride and encouragement in themselves and in others.

Consider how your students communicate to someone when that person fails. Do they mock, tease, laugh, and send other discouraging communication, either with words or with body language? Likewise, how do your students communicate to themselves, both externally and internally (self-talk) when they fail? Do you overhear your students mumbling to themselves, "I'm such a dummy. I can't do anything right!"? This type of communication (negative self-

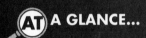

A GLANCE...

In this lesson on success and failure, you'll teach your students how to:

◆ praise and learn from other people's successes

◆ communicate self-pride when experiencing success

◆ encourage others and learn from their failures

◆ stick with difficult tasks, use positive self-talk, and request help to facilitate future success

talk) serves to discourage your students from pressing on to reach their goals.

Many students (several of whom are on our caseloads) get discouraged easily and quit, put themselves down, throw things, crumple up paper, pound their desks, or blame others for their failures. This communication lesson will help your students create a positive internal dialogue that will motivate them to stick with difficult tasks and/or request the help that will support their eventual success.

Vocabulary

self-talk: communicating to one's self internally and externally

flip the pancake: encouraging one's self to see the bright side of the situation when experiencing failure

Materials

paint (dark and light colors)

two large sheets of paper, poster board, or butcher paper

props necessary for any role plays you create

Springboard

Before you begin the lesson, place the two large sheets of paper in the front of the room with the paints. As the lesson unfolds, have your students use these materials to create Success and Failure Murals. Begin this communication lesson with the following activating questions:

Can anyone tell me what success is?

How many people like to succeed?

What are some things you have been successful at?

How does success make you feel?

What colors do you see when you think of success?

ur students talk about the colors that remind them of success, invite them to add a splash of this color to the Success Mural. They will create a mural of many different brilliant colors to remind them how bright and uplifting an experience success is. It has been my experience that the majority of students will choose bright colors, although any color is appropriate since it is merely the color that symbolizes a good feeling for each student. When the Success Mural is finished, you'll be ready to activate the students' prior knowledge about failure.

Who can tell me what failure is?

Can anyone talk about a time when they failed?

(Some of your classes may need to be prompted by hearing an example of when you or the classroom teacher experienced failure. You may be surprised at how honest and forthcoming your students will be about sharing their failures.)

Who likes to fail?

How does failing make you feel?

What colors do you see when you think of failure?

Ask your students to create a Failure Mural by adding the colors they see when they think of failure. Upon completion, place the two murals side-by-side and ask students to compare and contrast the different shades and the different feelings each experience brings.

Close the Springboard section of this CommunicationLab by explaining to your students, "Today in CommunicationLab, we're going to learn how to be good at failures." (You'll get some funny looks from students since most people want to avoid failure.) Reassure your students by explaining that as hard as we try, there will be times when we make mistakes or just don't succeed right away on our own. Your students will learn how to communicate to themselves and to others in a way that makes them feel (name some of the colors from the Success Mural), instead of (name some of the colors from the Failure Mural).

Warm Up

During this Warm Up Activity, you and the classroom teacher will role play to model helpful and hurtful communication when experiencing success and failure. By observing these role plays, your students will gain the vocabulary and necessary communication tools to effectively manage their own successes and failures.

Role Play 1
Pride/Learn from Others

In the first role play, select a student to play the role of a teacher who will instruct you and the classroom teacher (you will play the roles of children) to hop on your right foot three times. Both of you will experience success. One of you will boast about it, and the other will send a put-down, "You think you're so good. Watch this."

Following your role play, call "freeze" and ask your students to think about the following:

Who was successful?

How did we communicate about our own success?

How did we communicate about each other's success?

Was our communication helpful or hurtful? Why?

Now role play this situation again to illustrate how you can communicate pride in our own accomplishments without boasting. Further demonstrate how you can be proud for another person when they succeed, and how you can learn from others by either watching them or asking them for help.

Following the role play, explore your students' observations about your communication.

How was this kind of communication helpful?

How did it make everyone feel?

Role Play 2
Self-Talk and Flipping the Pancake

In this second role play, the student playing the role of the teacher will again ask you and the classroom teacher to hop on one foot, but this time you will both fail. One of you will verbally put yourself down by saying something like, "It figures. I never do anything right," while the other teacher will laugh and make fun of your failure. Call "freeze" and begin debriefing with your students about the communication they observed following your failure.

Who failed?

How did we communicate to ourselves?

Explain the concept of self-talk by pointing out that we have an internal dialogue with ourselves that either encourages or discourages us. For example, in the last role play you used negative self-talk.

Did my negative self-talk encourage or discourage us from succeeding?

How did we communicate to each other?

Was this helpful or hurtful? Why?

What colors did you see?

Role play the situation again to illustrate how we can communicate to ourselves and others to motivate and support success by using positive self-talk. For example, after experiencing failure you might say something like, "I'm gonna get it this time." Again, explore your students' observations about your communication and discuss the energy we derive from using positive self-talk following failure.

How did we communicate to ourselves and each other when we failed?

What colors did you see?

Suggest that in both the first and second role plays, you and the classroom teacher experienced failure, but because of the positive way you communicated to yourself and to each other, the experience wasn't so dark and gloomy.

Ricky, a second-grade student at Meadowbrook Elementary in Northbrook, Illinois, calls this "Flipping the Pancake." After observing the role play he said, "Ms. Pritchard, this is kind of like a pancake." Naturally, my first reaction was concern since I thought this was an unidentified language-impaired student with topic-maintenance problems. How in the world was he going to tie pancakes into this lesson? But then he explained, "On one side of the pancake, it's all dark, then you just communicate nicely to yourself and flip the pancake to the bright side." Well, you can bet I never needed to provide a language evaluation for Ricky since he was right on! In fact, now students throughout the United States remind each other to "Flip the Pancake" when they observe someone discouraged by failure. (Flipping the Pancake is much like reframing a situation to see the bright side.)

This is an example of how CommunicationLab can be tailored for your school. Begin the Lab by using the core vocabulary of the program. You'll soon be incorporating your students' and teachers' vocabulary and strategies into your program.

Success & Failure Role Plays

Success

In these role plays, you'll teach your students how to communicate with themselves and others when experiencing success. Through these role plays, your students will practice communicating pride and will learn from their friends' successes.

Creating Role Plays

Begin by recalling common successes that your students experience every day. Next, recall negative ways your students communicate to themselves and others when they succeed. (See the Role Play Suggestions.) You and the classroom teacher will then role play these situations for the students' observation.

For Older Students

Begin with the following brainstorm to help generate role plays.

What makes other people's success hard for you to handle? (for instance, bragging or putting someone down)

Then, invite a group of students to role play these situations. Use the suggested *Assessing Role Plays* questions to explore the importance of learning how to handle success. Then, have this same group role play these situations again to demonstrate better ways to handle success. Discuss the results.

Suggested Role Plays

◆ Boast when you complete the math problem first.

- Act embarrassed when your painting is chosen for first place in a contest.
- Tell a successful person he cheated.
- Tell a successful person that she was lucky, and you could do better.

Assessing Role Plays

Following the action, call "freeze" and think aloud with your students about the following:

How did we communicate with one another?

Does this kind of communication make you feel happy about another person's success? Why?

Problem Solving

Invite your students to re-role play by communicating in a more positive way when experiencing success. First, give them practice expressing pride about their own successful experiences. Next, provide them with opportunities to express admiration for a peer's success. Suggest that they ask the successful person to teach them how to be successful.

Failure

Role Play 1
Self-Talk and Flipping the Pancake

Create role plays to give your students practice using positive self-talk and the "Flipping the Pancake" technique to manage moments of failure. In this set of role plays, you'll play the role of a frustrated student who uses negative self-talk when experiencing failure.

For Older Students

Help your students create their own role plays by encouraging them to recall a time when they used negative self-talk after experiencing failure. Challenge a group of students to role play these situations for the group. Then, have this same group role play each situation again using the "Flipping the Pancake" technique and positive self-talk. Following each set of role plays explore the following:

How did they communicate with themselves?

Was this helpful? Why?

How did their communication make them feel?

Suggested Role Plays

Following failure, do one of the following:

- Bang on the desk.
- Crumple up your paper.
- Kick over a chair.
- Say, "I can't do anything right!"

Assessing Role Plays

Call "freeze" following the role play and discuss the following:

How did you handle failure?

Was this helpful or hurtful for your eventual success?

How could you have handled this differently?

Problem Solving

Invite a group of students to role play this situation again using the "Flipping the Pancake" technique and positive self-talk. Discuss how this kind of communication can empower us to persevere after failing to achieve success.

Role Play 2
Encouraging Others

Create role plays to help your students learn how to send encouragement when they observe someone's frustration from failing. In this set of role plays, the classroom teacher will play the part of a student who further aggravates the "frustrated failure."

For Older Students

Help your students create their own role plays with the following facilitative thoughts. "We've all talked about how it doesn't feel good to fail. Let's brainstorm to think of ways people communicate to us that make our failures feel worse." Invite students to role play these situations. Use the suggested *Assessing Role Plays* questions to initiate a discussion about encouraging others when they fail.

Challenge your students to role play these scenes again by communicating in a way that will empower someone to "Flip the Pancake" and pursue success.

Suggested Role Plays

After observing someone's failure, react as follows:

◆ Laugh at his failure.

◆ Point out her failure to another person.

◆ Tell him, "That's easy, anyone can do that!"

Assessing Role Plays

Following the role play, call "freeze" and ask your students the following:

is kind of communication make the person feel better or worse about his failure?

When you observe someone fail, what are some things you might do to make her feel better?

Problem Solving

Now your students are prepared to role play this situation again by responding to the person who failed in a way that will make him feel better. If your students need some suggestions, offer the following:

◆ Identify with the person's failure since it can happen to anyone.

◆ Encourage the frustrated person.

◆ Offer some suggestions about how to eventually succeed.

Notes

Wrap Up

"Today we learned that everyone experiences success and failure and that there are different ways to communicate to encourage yourself and others."

What can you do if you observe someone else succeed?

How can we communicate when we experience our own success?

How can you help a friend "Flip the Pancake" when you observe that she is discouraged by failure?

*What kind of self-talk can you use if you're
discouraged by failure?*

*How can I remind you to "Flip the Pancake"
when I observe that you're discouraged?*

Communication Challenge

Have your students review the Communication
Challenge from the previous week. Encourage
your students to talk about how they felt when
they sent you helpful criticism. Discuss any
changes in your teaching as a result of the
suggestions.

Then, challenge your students to help someone "Flip the Pancake" when they see a person
become discouraged because of failure.
Encourage your students to listen to their self-
talk during the day. Explain that if they catch
themselves using negative self-talk, they need
to try to "Flip the Pancake."

Classroom Carryover Activities

1. Proud Day

Declare a *Proud Day* for your classroom. During this day, challenge your students to notice and comment on others' successes; to learn from other people's strengths; to acknowledge their own accomplishments; and to share their pride with their teachers, parents, and friends. Bring your students together at the end of the day to talk about all the pride that was communicated throughout the day.

2. Flipping the Pancake

I have observed that students will use the "Flipping the Pancake" technique and positive self-talk when they can observe these concepts modeled and when they are encouraged by adults. Whenever you experience failure, use it as an opportunity to model positive self-talk for your students. For example, you might say, "I really need to 'Flip the Pancake.'" Likewise, when you observe students "Flipping the Pancake," make an immediate comment such as, "Good. You remembered to 'Flip the Pancake.'" Other students may need a reminder such as, "Looks like a good time to 'Flip the Pancake.'"

3. Positive Self-Talk

We often assign our students challenging tasks. Next time this occurs, urge your students to remember to use positive self-talk. When your students are engaged in the challenging activity, circulate around the room and comment positively on their body language. You might say, "It looks like you're using some positive self-talk." You may need to remind others to "Flip the Pancake."

Following this activity, ask your students which strategies they used. Which strategies encouraged them to stick with their challenging task? You may be surprised as your students begin creating strategies of their own that will give them the extra energy and confidence to persevere when the going gets tough.

Parent Lab

1. Receiving Praise

It's important for children to receive praise and feel proud. They may find it more comfortable and pleasing to be given praise in a "certain" way, like a smile or a pat on the back.

Initiate a conversation to brainstorm reasons family members praise each other. Discuss how the praise is sent. Then, have family members choose what they would like to be praised for and how they would like to be praised.

2. Sticking With Frustrating Tasks

Children can learn how to "stick with" frustrating tasks and cope with failures by watching how their parents manage similar situations. Create a "talk time" between parents and their children about coping with failure. Have them recall recent failures, how they felt, and how they coped.

Introduce the concept of positive self-talk. Think out loud with children as to when they might be able to use positive self-talk at home. Encourage parents to notice and reinforce their child's use of positive self-talk. Parents can also point out when they themselves use positive self-talk.

Dear Parents,

Success and failure were the topics of this week's CommunicationLab. Your child learned how to communicate pride for his success and for the success of others, as well as how to learn from his friends.

Don't be surprised if you hear your child saying things like, "Wow. That was terrific! How did you do that? Teach me." Use this opportunity to reinforce positive communication by praising your child for communicating pleasure for someone else's success.

When experiencing failure, learning how to communicate positively with ourselves and with others is equally important. In this week's lesson, your child learned how to use positive self-talk to encourage himself when he experiences failure. Ask your child to teach you about positive self-talk.

Children are constantly learning how to handle both success and failure by observing how family members handle these situations. It may be helpful for your whole family to discuss the different ways you encourage yourselves when the going gets tough. Likewise, discuss how you encourage each other. Share any personal encouragement or confidence boosters that you use to encourage your success and others. Together we can continue to give our children the communication tools they need to gain the confidence and courage to do their best!

We hope to see you next week on _____ from _____ to _____ to observe your child's participation in the final CommunicationLab.

Sincerely,

Lesson 10: Parent Review

We all know the frustration that results from having our teaching efforts sabotaged by our students' family members. On the other hand, we have observed how much faster our students learn and generalize new skills when we have the support of parents. Coordinating home and school efforts provides our students with a consistent program which encourages their success.

Unfortunately, gaining and maintaining parental support is often difficult because many parents have work schedules that conflict with their ability and desire to play an active role in their child's education. Your weekly letters to the parents not only gave them a convenient way to find out what their child was learning, but it also allowed you to offer suggestions about how they might further support the school's efforts to enhance their child's communication skills.

Now, at the close of CommunicationLab, you'll invite these parents to observe their child practicing these improved communication skills in the classroom. Understandably, many parents will be unable to attend. Therefore, I suggest videotaping the session so you can make this important information available to all of the parents.

To prepare for the parents' arrival, create an open space in the front of the room for role playing. Set chairs in a half circle surrounding the role-playing area so parents can easily view the action. Upon the parents' arrival, have the classroom teacher extend a warm welcome, thank the parents for their involvement and for supporting their child's communicative development, and introduce you, the communication teacher.

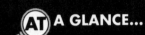 **A GLANCE...**

In this communication review session, you'll provide parents with the following opportunities to:

- hear and observe their child using the vocabulary from CommunicationLab

- observe how the teachers interact to facilitate good communicative behavior and cooperation

- observe their child's awareness of communication

- reinforce their commitment to improving their child's communication skills

Vocabulary

(See definitions in Chapter 5, Lesson 1, page 43)

observation

body language

listening

turn taking

the way

praise

criticism

success

failure

Materials

chalkboard

chairs

props necessary for any role plays you create

Springboard

Prior to this Parent Review Session, create a poster titled "What Do Good Communicators Do?" On this poster, list each of the communication skills that you covered during CommunicationLab. Place this poster in the front of the room so you can refer to it during the presentation.

To launch the Review Session and lay the groundwork for the program, ask your students the following:

What is communication?

Why is communication important at school? At home?

How does communication help us with our friendships?

Direct your students' attention to the list of communication skills on the poster. Review all the skills they learned during their participation in the Lab by reading aloud each skill from the list.

"Wow! That's a lot to remember when communicating. Today, you'll role play for your parents to show them what happens when people forget to use these good communication skills. Then, you'll show them how to problem solve to improve communication."

Your students are now ready to move into the role-playing section of this Lab. It has been my experience that some classes need a few minutes to warm up because they're nervous with their parents watching. If you sense this is the case, you may need to prompt your students by verbally narrating the first few role plays.

Role Plays for Younger Students

Creating Role Plays

Prior to the Review Session, create role plays that will illustrate each of the skills your class studied in CommunicationLab.

◆ Observation

◆ Body Language

◆ Listening

◆ Turn Taking

◆ The Way We Communicate

◆ Praise and Criticism

◆ Success and Failure

Role Playing Poor Communication

During the role plays, you and the classroom teacher will first model poor communication. For example, you'll demonstrate interrupting, poor eye contact, negative body language, etc.

Then the students will model good communication. You may have some classes that will be willing and able to participate in the role plays that demonstrate poor communication.

Assessing Role Plays

Following each role play, call "freeze" and ask your students the following questions:

Who wasn't a good communicator? Why?

What happened because of poor communication?

Role Playing Good Communication/Carryover Activities

Invite student volunteers to role play each situation again using improved communication skills. After each role play, give the parents some suggestions for carryover activities. For example, after a role play demonstrating the importance of observation skills, you might say, "In this role play, the children demonstrated how they can observe when someone is busy so they don't interrupt. If you notice that your child is observing more before communicating, be sure to praise him or her by saying something like, 'Thanks for noticing that I was busy. I can talk to you after I finish looking for my car keys.' If your child forgets to observe before he communicates, you may want to model this skill by observing when he is busy, and then saying something like, 'I observe that you're busy. When would be a good time to communicate?' "

Encourage parents to use the vocabulary of CommunicationLab as a vehicle to encourage good communication skills.

Helpful Tips

I've found that the students are more successful when I choose familiar role plays from previous classes. If your students have stage fright due to having an audience, you may need to narrate the first couple of role plays, telling your students exactly what to do and say. For example, you might say, "Then Mike looked at his mom and said he would throw out the garbage." Soon your students will warm up and will turn into the "hams" you've been enjoying these past nine weeks.

After completing the role plays, move to the Wrap Up section of the Lab.

Role Plays for Older Students

Creating Role Plays

Following the Springboard, invite your students to create role plays from this list of communication skills.

- ◆ Observation
- ◆ Body Language
- ◆ Listening
- ◆ Turn Taking
- ◆ The Way We Communicate
- ◆ Praise and Criticism
- ◆ Success and Failure

Help the students develop a role play for each skill by asking the following:

What happens when you don't take turns?

What happens when you don't use your observation skills?

What happens when you don't listen?

Role Playing Poor Communication/Good Communication

After a student describes what happens, invite a group of students to demonstrate first what happens when they don't use good communication, and then role play again to show what happens when they do use good communication.

Assessing Role Plays

Following each series of role plays, help your students debrief by having them discuss the differences in outcome because of poor and good communication.

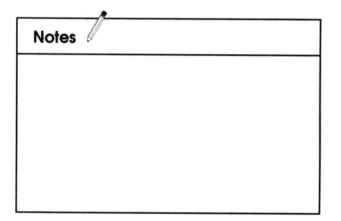

Notes

Wrap Up

Have the classroom teacher begin the Wrap Up by sharing her observations about the improved communication in the classroom. Citing specific examples of how students communicate differently because of CommunicationLab is a powerful reinforcement.

parents to share their observations about their children's improved communication since beginning CommunicationLab. You'll be surprised how forthcoming parents will be about the positive changes they've observed. If you receive no response from the parents, simply comment about your own observations. To conclude the Wrap Up, encourage the parents to communicate how proud they are of their children's accomplishments by applauding.

Communication Challenge

Challenge your students to continue their awareness of good communication. Have a discussion about what students can do in school and at home to continue practicing and improving their communication skills.

To conclude CommunicationLab, publicly thank the classroom teacher, students, and parents for all of their contributions. End the session with another round of applause that will fill your students with pride and positive energy to reinforce their commitment to improving their communication skills more and more each day!

Dear Parents,

Thank you for your participation and commitment to our Communication-Lab. Although our formal 10-week communication program is over, we'll continue to stress and reinforce the importance of using good communication skills at school and at home.

We hope that you'll join us in praising your child when you notice him using some of the skills learned in CommunicationLab. Please continue to provide your child with helpful reminders to recall and use these important skills.

We want to keep the lines of communication open between school and home. We encourage you to let us know how your family is reinforcing your child's good communication skills.

Thank you for your support!

Sincerely,

References

Andrews, J. R. and M. A. Andrews. *Family Based Treatment in Communicative Disorders: A Systemic Approach.* Sandwich, IL: Janelle Publications, 1990.

Dodge, E. P. *CommunicationLab 2.* East Moline, IL: LinguiSystems, Inc., 1994.

Dodge, E. P. *CommunicationLab Profile.* East Moline, IL: LinguiSystems, Inc., 1994.

Dodge, E. P. *Teachable Moments for Classroom Communication.* East Moline, IL: LinguiSystems, Inc., 1994.

Herer, G. "Inventing Our Future." <u>ASHA</u>, Vol. 31, 1989, pp. 35-37.

Ladd, G. W. "Having friends, keeping friends, making friends, and being liked by peers in the classroom: Predictors of children's early school adjustment." <u>Child Development</u>, Vol. 61, 1990, pp. 1081-1100.

Mallard, A. R. "Management of the young stutterer with parental involvement: a British-American project." <u>The College of Speech Therapists Bulletin</u>, Vol. 403, 1985, pp. 1-3.

Mallard, A. R., L. Rustin, and E. Pritchard. "Using the Elementary Classroom in a School-Based Service Delivery Model." Short Course presented at the ASHA Annual Convention, Seattle, WA, 1990.

Rustin, L., and A. Kuhr. *Social Skills and the Speech Impaired.* London, England: Taylor and Francis Ltd., 1989.

Ward, J.R. "Now Hear This." *IABC Communication World,* 1990, pp. 20-22.